MW01251668

show - 'Ka-posies' sarcoma
        kaposis sarcoma

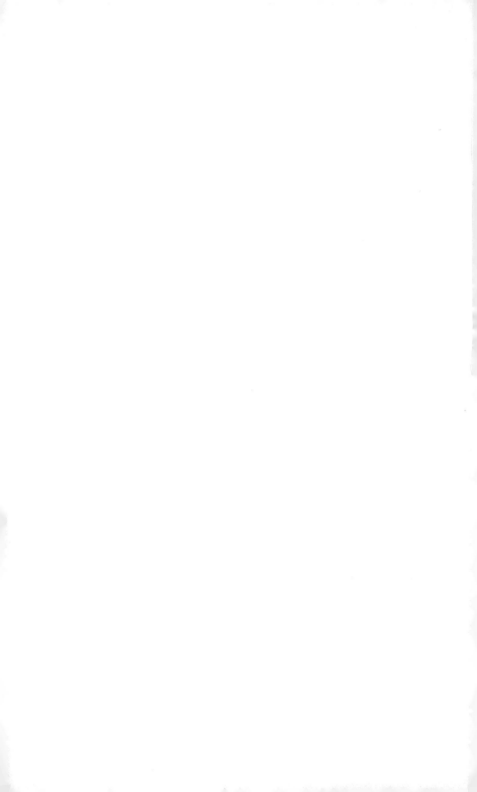

AIDS AND HIV-RELATED DISEASES

An Educational Guide for Professionals and the Public

[handwritten notes:]

Nureon p. 3?

= AZT =
  Azido-thyordine

= ZDV | AZT = anti-viral
  Crixivan   (protease inhibitor
              (blocks enzyme used
                by virus to replicate

p. 340 Nurone
= sexual exposure
  Male to Male   1.06 to 5.1
  male to female   1.05 - 1.23
  female to male   1.03 to 5.16

Needles
  sharing 67%

Mother to Infant
  25% → 8.3 (ZDV)

- Infected blood transfusion
  89.5%

AIDS AND HIV-RELATED DISEASES

An Educational Guide for Professionals and the Public

JOSH POWELL

Foreword by
Amy Bourdeau

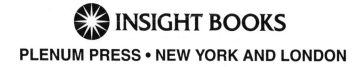 **INSIGHT BOOKS**

PLENUM PRESS • NEW YORK AND LONDON

Library of Congress Cataloging-in-Publication Data

Powell, Josh.
    AIDS and HIV-related diseases : an educational guide for
  professionals and the public / Josh Powell ; foreword by Amy
  Bourdeau.
        p.   cm.
    Includes bibliographical references and index.
    ISBN 0-306-45085-2
    1. AIDS (Disease)   2. HIV infections.   3. Health education.
  I. Title.
    [DNLM: 1. Acquired Immunodeficiency Syndrome--complications.
  2. AIDS-Related Opportunistic Infections.   WC 503.5 P884a 1996]
  RC607.A26P686   1996
  616.97'92--dc20
  DNLM/DLC
  for Library of Congress   96-29019
                                                                 CIP

The publisher and authors disclaim responsibility for any adverse
effects or consequences from the misapplication or injudicious
use of the information contained within this text. Never use any drugs, medical
procedures, or medical products without the consultation and instruction of
your physician. The publisher and author are not endorsing or promoting any
products within the confines of this work.

ISBN 0-306-45085-2

© 1996 Plenum Press, New York
Insight Books is a Division of Plenum Publishing Corporation
233 Spring Street, New York, N.Y. 10013-1578

An Insight Book

10 9 8 7 6 5 4 3 2 1

Foreword

In recent years, there has been increased public entreaty to develop potential therapies more rapidly for many life-threatening diseases for which there are no effective medical treatments. Many patient-advocacy groups have had some success in expediting the release of new drugs from ongoing clinical trials; thus, the incentive and motivation to put pressure on the research community continues to grow. Patient-advocacy groups establish strong and oftentimes very powerful voices through demonstrations, powerful publicity tactics, and multiple interactive media. As the "information superhighway" continues to grow, it allows patient-support groups extensive access to countless individuals throughout the United States and the world. Circulating personal accounts of an afflicted individual's suffering serves to fuel the fire in terms of public support. These groups have evolved into extremely powerful assemblages by sheer virtue of their size and subsequently have met with success in influencing researchers, the pharmaceutical and biotechnology industries, and, ultimately, the division of government that sets forth the regulations governing the release of new drugs into the market.

Advocacy groups place enormous pressures on drug developers to accelerate the development (and therefore the release) of drugs, as well as expanded access to drugs under investigation. These pressures have generated many changes in the architecture of drug-development guidelines. Although it is human nature to empathize with the plight of patients who endure the massive burden of a life-threatening disease for which there exists little or no therapy, it remains the responsibility of the developer and the governing agency to assess objectively the safety of a potentially therapeutic compound before it is administered to a patient. Despite the urgencies expressed by activist groups, it remains the ultimate responsibility of the developer and the regulatory agencies to characterize any and all safety issues that may accompany the administration of compounds under development. The evolution of regulatory agencies was such that each developing compound would be fully understood before its marketability was assessed. The Food and Drug Administration, through complex trial and error, has arrived at a set of guidelines for the development of new drugs. These regulations outline a commonsense approach to bringing new therapies to market. In terms of patient health, a compound must have an acceptable safety profile before it can be administered to a patient whose health is already compromised. Those patients who, on their own accord, accept the responsibility and potential consequences of taking an uncharacterized compound may ultimately be putting themselves at an even greater risk than that imposed by their disease.

This is not to say that agencies that regulate drug development should not grant special consideration and accelerated review of those therapies that are most in demand, but rather that as much information as is required and necessary should be in hand before a drug is allowed into circulation. Taking away researchers' ability to regulate the characterization of their compounds takes away their ability to make appropriate decisions about the therapeutic relevance of the drugs. Science and its advancement may ultimately suffer because of efforts to satisfy the demands of the advocacy groups.

This book attempts to summarize, describe, and illustrate many of the clinical manifestations of diseases that are attributable to HIV and cause a diagnosis of AIDS. The relatively recent onset of the HIV/AIDS epidemic in the United States demands that a fundamental instructional resource be made available for use in clinical, academic, and private settings. Due to the large number of disorders associated with AIDS and the social disdain at present associated with the virus, it becomes essential that a comprehensive description of these disorders be outlined for those who may be called upon to instruct on the subject. This book is written to be understood not only by clinicians but also by the layperson who has little or no background in science. It is the author's intent to produce a practical desktop resource useful to all basic and clinical researchers interested in the complications surrounding HIV/AIDS-related diseases. The chapters that follow provide a comprehensive and discernible description of the disease that will be useful over a range of professions.

Because of the ever-increasing incidence of AIDS, it is essential that its dynamics (i.e., the progression of the virus and the events following contraction) be addressed both in the classroom and in the realm of social services. The virus has become so widespread that people are not truly safe unless they understand how they can protect themselves. The following text offers ideas and commentary on useful ways to educate and inform people of all ages about HIV/AIDS. It serves as a very basic tool for understanding and explaining the dynamics of the disease to children, teens, and adults. The author presents a very real and compassionate commentary on the problems that are inherent in the homosexual population and those that may arise when educating family members of those infected with the virus. Actual case histories are presented as reference tools to illustrate the broad scope of the virus, and the cases are described in understandable and practical dialogue. The references and examples used in this book are real, which in itself will convince the reader of the indiscriminate nature of the virus.

Unique problems arise for those who are both young and homosexual and in addition HIV-positive. The author's own experiences coupled with his clinical experience allow him to discuss unique problems associated with being HIV-positive in such a way as to enlighten both educators and students. The most wonderful thing about this book, however, is that it is a dramatically genuine and honest description of many of the sociodynamic implications that go along with being HIV-positive in contemporary society. It is not enough to be sympathetic to the patient. It is important that HIV/AIDS patients be comforted and consoled, but they and their families need more. They need to understand the disease and its components in order to be better prepared for what lies ahead.

I am pleased to say that I have known the author for well over a decade now and was honored to have been asked to write this foreword. His sincere dedication to his studies and the verity that the profits from this book will go to further AIDS education is proof positive that the author is the most genuine of researchers. The book represents the author's best effort at compiling both his personal accounts and information gathered from other sources. It will, I hope, prove illuminating for all those working in the field in the years ahead.

AMY R. BOURDEAU, B.S.

Preclinical Research Associate
Department of Toxicology, Amgen, Inc.
Los Angeles, California

Acknowledgments

This book could not have been written without the support of the many men and women who allowed me access to their lives and shared with me their experiences living with HIV. Their generosity was, and continues to be, an inspiration.

I would also like to thank my mother and father, Dorothy and Joseph, my sisters, Lucy and Leah, and my brother, Seth, for their support and patience.

Finally, this book could not have been completed without the help of Joyce Timmons, Michele Samal, Margaret Walsh, Esq., Ellen Ewasic, and Ray DiMarco.

Contents

Introduction

This book is about the disease called AIDS and society's response to it. The disease itself is something that could have come out of a science fiction novel: A slow, lurking virus eventually causes an agonizing death. Groups of people fight a government that treats them as lepers. AIDS, though, is not a fiction. For some, like me, who were growing up when AIDS was first being seen, it is a reminder that there was once a time when there was no deadly virus that might come along as a result of a sexual encounter. For some people, AIDS is real, and when it is real it can be hell on earth.

I first started working with people who had AIDS in 1988 while I was employed at a drug rehabilitation center. At the time, I thought AIDS was a disease that some injection drug users contracted, but in upstate New York AIDS was still something of a rumor. I remember clearly when AIDS made an appearance in my life. I was at a staff meeting, and there was talk about a client who took an HIV test and got a positive result. I knew this man well; he was my age, and I had many conversations with him. I felt very sad, and past the sadness, there was a fear that this was the start of an onslaught. AIDS was very new to me, and it scared me. I thought that I might "catch" the virus from a client. I was told that this was not going to happen because a person needed to have direct contact with an infected person's blood. But I was not so sure; I thought that the science was new, and that this mysterious virus, this thing, might be able to infect me in a different way—an unknown but easy way. It all became a moot point for me. I was working alone one night at the rehab. I was sitting at my desk when a client ran into the office in a panic. She told me that another woman upstairs in the women's room had just passed out and was bleeding through the nose. I ran up the stairs and found this woman, whom I will call Mary, on the floor. Mary's apparent cocaine use was so profound that the inside of her nose had started to break apart, causing severe bleeding. She was starting to gag on her own blood, and I knew that she needed to be brought to a sitting position so that the blood would not fall into the windpipe. I held her upright while I told the other client to go and call for help. By the time that the paramedics arrived, I was covered in this woman's blood.

When I went to work again, I was told that this woman was HIV positive. I did not contract HIV from this experience, but I did have to go through the tests, and I wondered for six months if I might have HIV. After that experience, AIDS simply became a more pronounced issue for me, and no longer seemed far away.

As a human service worker, I was amazed at how AIDS became an enormous issue to those who work "in the field." I was amazed at the treatment that many of these men and women said that they endured. This was not what being human is about. The people who had this disease were not only suffering from an awful condition, but also were slammed by the press, politicians, and conservative groups. The things that I read about AIDS usually had to do with either the disease itself, or about the person who had the disease and how he or she became infected. There seemed to be little information available that explained the disease, how it became so widespread, and why some groups seemed to get it more than others.

I started to explain these concepts to others, as my studies brought me closer to a better understanding of AIDS and HIV. While reading and taking courses that helped me to understand the human body and the way that AIDS affects it, there was something missing. AIDS was not to me a disease that could be understood without talking to those who had AIDS about the disease and what it is like to have it.

As part of an academic project, I began to talk to people who had AIDS. I arranged to speak with them by posting notices on bulletin boards, contacting agencies that worked with people who had AIDS, and running classified ads. I was not prepared for what was about to happen. People had something to say about having HIV and about the treatment that they received from health and human service organizations, employers, friends, family, and society as a whole. The world that they see is often a hostile one, and not just because of HIV. Those people most likely to be infected with HIV are not those whom polite society likes to talk about, help out, and support. For these people—gay men, injection drug users, and sex trade workers—prejudice is a part of their everyday lives.

I spoke with over 220 people who either were HIV-positive or had AIDS. After finishing the interviews, I was left with the feeling that I had been off to war. I saw young men and women who were at a point in life where they should have been considering buying homes and raising families instead of fearing certain death. There were valiant heroes and loved ones left behind to mourn the dead, but this war is lost every day as a man dies in New York, and another in Miami. When a son, brother, father, mother, or friend dies, the survivors face a world of such profound emotional impoverishment that life is often divided into two phases: before and after AIDS.

The "war" against AIDS is won every time a person makes an effort to prevent its spread, thus preventing the pain and loss that AIDS brings to him and those who care about him; every time a new drug is invented that helps keep a person infected with HIV healthy; and every time a kind gesture is extended to understand and support the people who survive with the disease.

1

Understanding HIV and Its Effect on the Immune System

AIDS is an acronym for *acquired immunodeficiency syndrome*, a disease characterized by the slow demise of the body's immune system. The agent thought to cause AIDS is the *human immunodeficiency virus*, commonly called HIV. The terms AIDS and HIV are not synonymous. AIDS refers to the end stages of an HIV infection, stages that are characterized by the presence of certain diseases. A diagnosis of AIDS means that a person has HIV, plus either one or more of 26 opportunistic infections or a T-cell count below 200 per cubic millimeter (mm^3). (T cells are the cells that mediate immunity.)

To understand AIDS and its impact on the body, it is necessary to understand the immune system and how HIV interrupts the role of this system in disease prevention. As the name suggests, the immune system is not a single structure that protects the body from disease. Rather, it is the functions of many cells, organs, and processes acting collectively to protect the body from a host of threats that can cause disease.

The Human Immune System

All living organisms are continuously exposed to substances that are capable of causing them harm. Most organisms protect themselves against such substances in more than one way—with physical barriers, for example, or with chemicals that repel or kill invaders. Man has not only these types of general protective mechanisms, but also a more advanced protective system that is referred to as the *immune system*. The immune system is a complex network of organs containing cells that recognize pathogens, or infectious agents, and destroys them. The term *pathogen* is a broad one that is used to denote a disease-causing substance. Common pathogens usually fall into one of three categories: bacteria, viruses, or funguses and parasites.

Bacteria

Bacteria are unicellular organisms that have a cell wall surrounding a cellular membrane. These organisms can cause disease when they enter tissues and release toxins. Such toxins are often carried throughout the body in the bloodstream. Examples of bacteria are streptococcus and chlamydia. Most bacterial infections can be treated with antibiotics.

Viruses

Viruses are very different from bacteria in that they are not living creatures. A virus is a piece of nucleic acid with a protein coating. Viruses do not carry out metabolic functions because they lack the ability to synthesize protein and produce energy. For this reason, viruses need other cells to reproduce. They command a host cell's biochemical machinery to use the viral nucleic acid as a program for the cell to follow. It is thus analogous to the way a disk puts a computer to use. A program disk without the computer is useless. Once the disk is placed in the computer, the disk has the ability to run the computer. The same can be said of a virus's ability to run a cell. The effect that the virus has on a cell it has infected is dependent upon the type of virus it is and on what type of cell it has infected. The end result of a viral infection can range from something as mild as a cold to something as deadly as cancer.

Funguses and Parasites

Funguses and parasites are organisms that feed off the body. Examples of these are worms, malaria pathogens, and athlete's foot fungus.

Although there are many potentially harmful pathogens, no pathogen can invade or attack all organisms because a pathogen's ability to cause harm requires a susceptible victim, and not all organisms are susceptible to the same pathogens. This difference is illustrated by the fact that HIV does not infect animals such as dogs and cats; likewise, man does not fall victim to canine distemper or feline leukemia.

Pathogens enter the body in a variety of ways: through cuts and abrasions in the skin, by absorption through the mucous membranes (nose, mouth, rectum, vagina, and urethra), and by ingestion. The largest organ in the body, the skin, is the first barrier to disease. The outer layers of the skin are rich in keratin, a substance that seals the epidermis (the outermost layer of the skin) by providing a waterproof barrier that keeps most pathogens from entering the body. When the skin is damaged, immunity is compromised. For example, the gravest threat to a severely burned person is that of infection resulting from the extensive damage to the skin.

Unlike the surface of the body, the openings in the body (the mouth, nose, anus, and genitalia) do not have an outer layer of keratinized epithelial cells, but are lined with cells that produce thick mucus that traps particles and keeps them from entering the body. But these physical barriers that the body employs to prevent infection are not always completely effective. Particles bypass the barriers by means of scratches, cuts, blisters, and other openings in the skin. Once a particle has made its way into the body, the immune system must take action in order to prevent disease. This is accomplished through a complicated collaboration among the cells that comprise the cellular immune system.

The Cell

Cells are often referred to as the basic building blocks of life. Cells carry out many functions, such as transporting nutrients, water, and enzymes; causing movement; conducting nervous impulses; and still others that protect the body. Life begins with a single cell dividing over and over to form an embryo. Once a zygote (an early embryo) has reached a certain stage in development, its cells begin to specialize. Specialization is the process by which cells differentiate and begin to assume specific roles needed to sustain life. Figure 1.1 shows a typical cell.

Cellular functions are carried out when the cell receives instructions from its nucleus. Inside the nucleus is a structure called the nucleolus. In the nucleolus, genetic material "expresses" or "defines" commands that the cell must execute. The genetic code, which resides in all cells that have a nucleus, contains all the necessary information to create an identical being. Note, however, that although the cell may have the appropriate information to create another being, it still follows its own particular path and function.

The genetic code is composed of many bits of genetic information called genes. Genes are composed of the protein deoxyribonucleic acid (DNA), which consists of four different types of protein: thymine (T), adenine (A), cytosine (C), and guanine (G). These proteins are often called base proteins, and are arranged in groups of three, called codons. Hundreds of codons grouped together form a gene, and these genes are collectively grouped on a chromosome. Figure 1.2 shows the arrangement of genetic matter in the cell.

The chromosome is a long strand of DNA shaped like a double helix. The placement of genes on the chromosome is very

The Cell

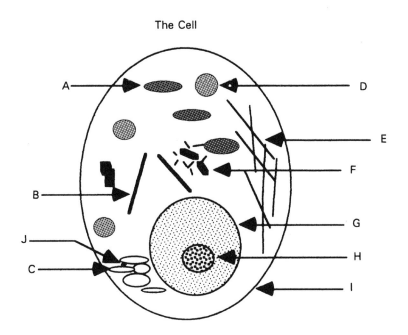

A. Mitochondria

B. Centromere

C. Golgi apparatus

D. Lysosome

E. Microfilaments

F. Centioles

G. Nucleus

H. Nucleolus

I. Cell membrane

J. Endoplasmic Reticulum

FIGURE 1.1. Schematic representation of a cell containing the various organelles that are common to most cells in the human body.

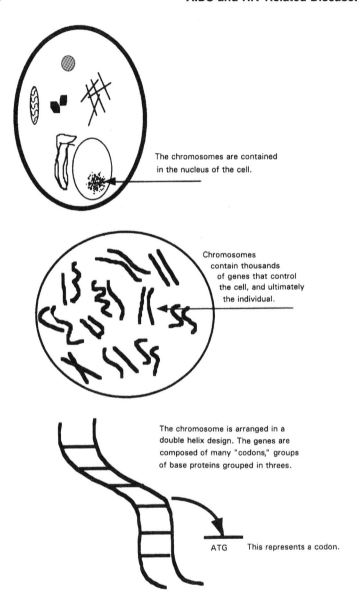

The chromosomes are contained
in the nucleus of the cell.

Chromosomes
contain thousands
of genes that control
the cell, and ultimately
the individual.

The chromosome is arranged in a
double helix design. The genes are
composed of many "codons," groups
of base proteins grouped in threes.

ATG   This represents a codon.

ATGATGATGATGATGATGATGATGATGATGATGATGATGATGATGAT

This is a gene.

FIGURE 1.2. Simplified cell illustrating the genetic matter in the cell.

important. It can be compared to a combination lock having many possible combinations, but only one that opens the lock. In the body, it is imperative that the right combination be used. Furthermore, with the lock, an incorrect combination will mean only that the lock will not open. In the body, an incorrect combination can cause disease, such as cancer. If a gene is positioned incorrectly, the results can be catastrophic. Genetic errors can happen for no apparent reason, or from exposure to certain substances. The genetic makeup of some cells can be altered by exposure to extreme doses of radiation, by environmental pollutants such as heavy metals, and by viruses such as HIV.

Cellular Immunity

Humoral innate immunity refers to the substances found in body fluids—for example, the blood (the term *humoral* comes from the Latin word *humor*, "a body fluid")—that interfere with the growth of pathogens or can clump them together so that they are eliminated from the body. The second component, called *cellular* innate immunity, is carried out by cells called *phagocytes* that ingest and degrade, or "eat," pathogens, and by so-called *natural killer cells* that destroy certain cancerous cells.

The human immune system also has *adaptive* immunity, which can recognize and destroy specific substances. The defensive reaction of the adaptive immune system is called the *immune response*. Any substance capable of generating this response is called an *antigen*, or immunogen. Antigens are not the foreign microorganisms and tissues themselves; they are substances—such as toxins or enzymes—in the microorganisms or tissues that the immune system considers foreign. Immune responses are normally directed against the antigen that provoked them and are said to be antigen-specific. *Specificity* is one of the two properties that distinguish adaptive immunity from innate immunity; the other is called *immunologic memory*. Immunologic memory is the ability of the adaptive immune system to mount a stronger and more effective immune response against an antigen after its first encounter with that antigen through a completed reaction—the immune response.

The immune response is marshaled by cells called *leukocytes*, often referred to as *white cells*. Leukocytes make up less than 5% of the blood. The other components of the blood are red blood cells (hemocytes), which deliver oxygen to tissues throughout the body (45% of the blood is comprised of these cells); platelets, the cells responsible for the clotting properties of blood; and plasma, which is the clear fluid portion of the blood that contains inorganic salts, foods, gases, enzymes, extracellular corpuscles, and various hormones (50% of the blood is comprised of plasma).

Leukocytes can be subdivided into five basic categories: neutrophils, eosinophils, basophils, monocytes, and lymphocytes. Neutrophils, eosinophils, and basophils are classified as polymorphonuclear granulocytes. These cells have a multilobed nucleus and many granules that are bound to membrane material inside the cell.

A monocyte is larger than a polymorphonuclear granulocyte. It has fewer granules that the others and has a larger U-shaped nucleus.

The final type of white cell is the lymphocyte. This is a large cell that, like the monocyte, has a large nucleus, but contains less cytoplasm (the intracellular fluid that can be viewed as the cell's blood).

All of these cells are produced in bone marrow, which comprises the center of long bones such as the sternum and femur.

Nonspecific Immune Responses

A nonspecific immune response is one that attacks any foreign particle. The attacking agents, those that do not discriminate between disease-carrying and non-disease carrying particles, are neutrophils. Neutrophils are the white blood cells that are most numerous, and they are destroyed in the greatest number because they are the first to arrive at the site of an infection. The cells that are killed in the process of fighting an infection make up what is commonly called *pus*.

The neutrophils have many sacs, called *lysosomes* or *granules*, containing enzymes that are released to attack and destroy foreign cells and particles.

The monocyte is the largest circulating cell in the body. Like the neutrophil, the monocyte is a cell of the nonspecific immune system. The monocytes are in the bloodstream for only a few days, after which they migrate to various organs and develop into macrophages. The macrophages destroy infectious particles in a very different way than do the enzyme-releasing neutrophils: A macrophage surrounds a particle and digests it. This process is called *phagocytosis*.

Specific Immune Response

While the nonspecific immune responses are effective in combating foreign particles, what must be remembered is that many organisms are designed to survive by living off another system. That is, many organisms are parasitic and are designed to be able to penetrate the body's defenses. There is a competition between the processes by which the body seeks to maintain and defend itself (referred to as *homeostasis*) and those by which a foreign organism seeks to overwhelm the body's defenses and thereby gain the means of its own survival. The body has to be vigilant against the many threats posed by the world, but the slow evolutionary process that has enabled man to accomplish so much has not benefitted our species alone. Microorganisms, parasites, viruses, and other pathogens have also had millions of years to hone their abilities to infiltrate and survive. To combat many of these pathogens, the body has devised a way of recognizing and destroying specific substances before they cause disease. This process of recognition and destruction is called a *specific immune response*.

Lymphocytes, like all white blood cells, are created in the

bone marrow. After leaving the bone marrow, they enter either the thymus or the lymph tissue (such as tonsils and lymph nodes). Depending on where they go after they leave the bone marrow, they become T cells or B cells. The T cells are those that mature in the thymus.

Two major classes of T cells are produced in the thymus: helper T cells and cytotoxic, or killer, T cells. Helper T cells secrete molecules called *interleukins* (abbreviated IL) that promote the growth of both B and T cells. The interleukins secreted by lymphocytes are also called *lymphokines*. The interleukins secreted by monocytes and macrophages are called *monokines*. Some ten different interleukins are known: IL-1, IL-2, IL-3, IL-4, IL-5, IL-6, IL-7, interferon, lymphotoxin, and tumor necrosis factor. Each interleukin has complex biological effects.

Cytotoxic T Cells

Cytotoxic T cells destroy cells infected with viruses and other pathogens and may also destroy cancerous cells. Cytotoxic T cells are also called *suppressor lymphocytes* because they regulate immune responses by suppressing the function of helper cells so that the immune system is active only when necessary.

The receptors of T cells are "trained" to recognize fragments of antigens that have been combined with a set of molecules found on the surfaces of all cells. These molecules are called *major histocompatibility complex* (MHC) molecules. As T cells circulate through the body, they scan the surfaces of body cells for the presence of foreign antigens that have been picked up by the MHC molecules. This function is called *immune surveillance*.

B Cells

The B cells are produced in the lymph tissues. The B cell is different from the T cell in that it can change into a plasma cell during an immune response. During the immune response, macrophages give information to the T cells about the invader. The T cells, while fighting the infection, will also give the B cells information about the pathogen. In response, the B cells transform into plasma cells.

A plasma cell contains more cytoplasm and is larger than a B cell. In this cytoplasmic environment, there are additional ribosomes (which are often referred to as the powerhouse of the cell because they synthesize proteins and are responsible for energy production). These ribosomes produce a special protein, called an *antibody*, that is specific to the antigen that is causing the infection. The antibody combines with the antigen and disables it. After the antigen is destroyed, the B cells no longer transform into plasma cells. Instead, they produce what are called *memory cells*. These memory cells are specific to the infection that caused the response and can be used only to fight it. For example, the presence of memory cells evoked by the chicken pox virus protects only against future infection by that virus.

A third class of lymphocytes is called *natural killer* (NK) cells. The origin of these cells is still unclear to scientists, and their role in the immune response is not fully known.

Understanding what composes the immune system is only part of understanding AIDS. It is very important to understand how the immune system functions and what happens when it fails.

Understanding the Function of the Immune System in Disease Control

When a disease-causing substance enters the body, it comes into contact with thousands of cells. Each cell that is native to the body is encased in protein that the body can recognize as being native. If the body's cells cannot recognize the new particle as native, then they will attack this particle. Usually, it is the neutrophils that invade the particle and destroy it. There is often inflammation at the site of the infection. This inflammation is caused by the large numbers of neutrophils that arrive at the site of infection The neutrophils kill the invader by releasing the enzymes contained in their cytoplasmic interiors. This process is termed *nonspecific cell-mediated immune response.*

Viral Infections

Once inside the body, a virus will search for a cell with a nucleus in order to replicate, using the cell's ability to synthesize proteins. Once this occurs, the virus is able to proliferate and infect other cells. The process continues in this fashion until the host dies or is able to keep the virus in check.

There is as yet no cure for any viral infection; the standard treatment for a viral infection is a vaccine, which stimulates the body into producing antibodies against that specific virus. Often, the vaccination is effected by introducing a killed or weakened strain of the virus into the body. The vaccination does not prevent or cure the disease; rather, it stimulates the body to respond to the antigen quickly, thus preventing the person from becoming sick. Aside from vaccines, viruses must run their course, with resulting fevers, aches, pains, and other discomfort. Some viruses, such as rabies, are extraordinarily lethal and kill victims swiftly. Others, such as herpes, recur frequently; medication can sometimes help to ease the symptoms, but there is no cure per se for the infection.

HIV: The Virus Thought to Cause AIDS

The human immunodeficiency virus (HIV) is a *retrovirus*, which refers to the type of virus that is made of RNA instead of DNA proteins. With the aid of an enzyme called *reverse transcriptase*, a retrovirus produces an analog of itself. This analog is a DNA form of the virus that implants itself into the genetic material of the commandeered cell. Once this implantation occurs, the cell follows HIV's DNA program, which turns the infected cell into a virus-producing factory. Necessary cell functioning is impaired, and eventually the virus kills the cell. HIV identifies a host cell by the protein on its surface. It has a particular affinity for CD4 protein. The cells that have this protein are T cells, specifically CD4 lymphocytes.

Once HIV is in the body, an immune-response occurs and antibodies are eventually produced. The virus is now sequestered within the T cell, one of the very cells that mediate immunity. Since the virus is inside the cell, the cell cannot be recognized as anything but a T cell. The T cell thus acts not only as a factory for HIV productions, but also as a Trojan horse that conceals HIV. When the infection first occurs, there is a massive fight between HIV and the body's immune system. A person who is infected with HIV might at this point feel the effects of this fight. Symptoms might include fever, chills, and other indicators that resemble the flu.

The process by which HIV subverts the body's specific immune response is illustrated in Figures 1.3–1.6.

Case Study 1.1

Chris is a 23-year-old gay male. He is currently being treated at a clinic for observation of his HIV status, which is positive. Chris has been infected with the virus for 2 years. He is currently experiencing no difficulties with his health. Two years ago, Chris had a serious cold with fevers, fatigue, cough, and diarrhea. It is thought that these symptoms suggested the time period in which Chris developed his HIV infection.

The average individual infected with HIV can expect a period of 5–7 years of relatively good health, after which the virus begins to reproduce itself at a rate greater than the body can respond to. This reproduction not only causes a rise in the amount of virus in the body, but also keeps the T cells from completing their task—that is, to mediate and assist in an immune response.

When the body stops protecting itself from opportunistic infections, the patient crosses the line from being HIV-antibody-positive to having AIDS.

Understanding AIDS as a Disease of Diseases

An AIDS diagnosis is meant to describe a state of health, specifically the poor state, on the continuum of an HIV infection.

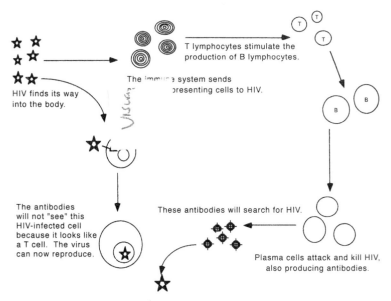

FIGURE 1.3. Diagram illustrating the immune system's response to an antigen, proceeding from recognition of foreign particles in the body to the point at which an antibody is produced.

The diseases that people with AIDS suffer with are called *oppor-tunistic infections*. These diseases must be explained individually if one is to fully grasp the concept of AIDS as a disease characterized by the presence of other diseases. Because of the nature of these diseases, AIDS renders its victims prey to increasingly severe physical torment and consequent psychological debilitation.

Chronic Fatigue Syndrome

Recently recognized, though not well understood, is a disease called chronic fatigue syndrome (CFS). Symptoms of CFS include fatigue; neurological, joint, and muscle problems; and general impairment of functioning. Accompanying illness may tempo-rarily abate spontaneously; accordingly, the person may have

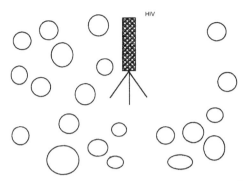

FIGURE 1.4. HIV travels through the body looking for a host cell to invade and eventually take over so that it can produce copies of itself.

"flare-ups" alternating with periods during which the disease is in remission and the person feels perfectly fine. Some research indicates that CFS occurs along with an impairment in the activity of NK cells.

Case Study 1.2

Susan is a 42-year-old woman who was diagnosed with CFS 3 years ago. "I started to feel a little run-down, just sort of tired a lot of the time. After a few weeks of feeling kind of tired, I decided to go to my doctor for a checkup. He said that there was nothing wrong with me. And I was pretty sure that he was right. I was tired, that's all. I also work a pretty hard shift at a hospital and thought that maybe I was just internalizing a lot of the things that I saw on the ward.

"It was three weeks after I saw that doctor that I was just too tired to get out of bed. I mean, I really could not get out of bed. It is like when you are deprived of sleep for days and then you get the chance to sleep, but after about five minutes someone tries to get you up, and you can't. That's what this is like."

Coccidioidomycosis

Coccidioidomycosis is a fungal infection caused by inhaling the spores of *Cocciodioides immitis*, which is commonly found in

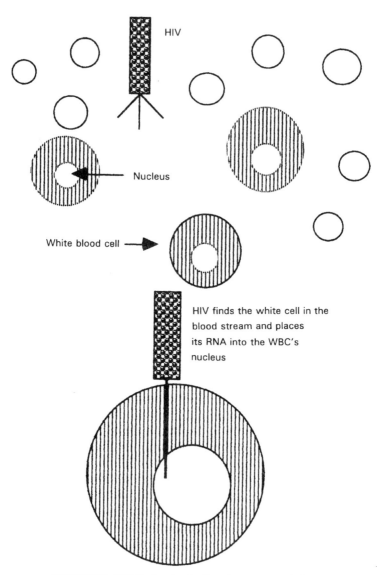

FIGURE 1.5. HIV finds a host cell and attempts to infect it.

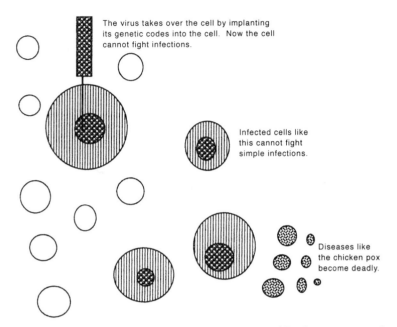

The virus takes over the cell by implanting its genetic codes into the cell. Now the cell cannot fight infections.

Infected cells like this cannot fight simple infections.

Diseases like the chicken pox become deadly.

FIGURE 1.6. HIV takes over the cell and leaves it incapable of recognizing and fighting other diseases. Thus unchecked, even common diseases such as chicken pox become deadly.

the southwestern United States, Mexico, and Latin America. It is also known as California disease, valley fever, desert rheumatism, and San Joaquin Valley fever. Travelers have become infected and not exhibited symptoms for a long time thereafter. The reason for the seemingly long dormancy period between exposure and disease is not known. There are two forms of the disease. The first is a self-limiting respiratory infection. The symptoms may resemble bronchitis and include fever, shortness of breath, unproductive cough, weight loss, and fatigue. They may vary in severity or resolve themselves only to reappear.

The second form of this disease is progressive coccidioidomycosis, which is virulent and severe if it is unchecked or if it occurs in the presence of HIV. Its symptoms may include anemia, allergy stimulation, skin problems, and inflammation of veins. There may be central nervous system (CNS) involvement as well.

Cryptococcosis

Cryptococcosis is caused by the fungus *Cryptococcus neoformans*, which is commonly found in dust or soil that has been contaminated by bird droppings. It is readily transmittable and fairly common in people with AIDS (PWAs). It enters the body through the respiratory tract and causes inflammation of meninges (the membranous coverings of the brain and spinal cord). The CNS is commonly involved. Without timely and aggressive treatment, the disease can be extremely dangerous. Symptoms include the appearance of CNS lesions, diffuse meningitis, cryptococcal meningitis, meningeal granulomas, soft areas, tissue destruction, and neuralgia.

Common symptoms are headaches, blurred vision, confusion, inappropriate speech or behavior, agitation, stiff or aching neck, and fever. Over the passage of time, the lungs, skin, or kidneys may be affected. Cryptococcosis also may cause coma. It is detected by a sputum test, which may reveal budding yeast with clear capsular matter around buds, and pus or other secretions. In the case of PWAs, a fungus culture from a blood sample is often performed. A lumbar puncture or spinal tap reveals a high lymphocyte count and an abnormally high protein level; a CAT scan may be needed to check for brain lesions.

Kaposi's Sarcoma

Kaposi's sarcoma (KS) is a cancer or neoplasm of connective tissue that supports blood vessels. It is sometimes referred to as a "skin cancer" because it produces visible lesions beneath the skin. It may also appear elsewhere, such as in the mouth, throat, and organs. It appears as spotted areas of pink, purple, or brown nodes or plaques that are irregular in shape and range in size from 3 to 40 mm (approximately 0.1 to 1.6 inches). These spots may grow and darken, or grow together at the edges. There is no pain associated with them.

Lymphadenopathic KS spreads quickly through the inner organs such as the lymph glands and the gastrointestinal (GI) tract. In the GI tract, KS appears as pigmented plaques or nodules. These lesions may be red, purple, or blue; flat or raised; and solitary or multiple. Early-stage or tentative KS lesions may be removed by laser surgery and treated by radiotherapy or by a lightly administered chemotherapy agent.

KS may also occur in the nose or rectum or on the eyelids. It is by nature proliferative. KS may be aggressive and radiation therapy may be required. However, treatment can be complicated by the rapid onset of severe inflammation of mucous membranes and often may have to be interrupted.

Cryptosporidiosis

Cryptosporidiosis is an infection caused by cryptosporidium, a protozoan parasite found in the intestines of animals. It is transmitted by direct contact with feces of infected animals or persons or by ingestion of contaminated food or water. This disorder attacks the intestines and after 5–15 days causes severe (explosive) diarrhea and abdominal cramps, which may last for 10–12 days, then temporarily abate.

Other possible symptoms include fever, nausea, vomiting, and weight loss. In HIV-positive persons, however, onset may be more gradual and the symptoms more severe. For example, an individual may evacuate more than 15 liters of fluid daily.

The illness may abate for extended periods of time, then reappear. Diagnosis is made by the presence of acid-fast oocysts in multiple stool cultures. (Stools of infected persons or animals are highly infectious.)

Symptomatic persons (those displaying signs of a specific disease) must drink plenty of fluids, maintain a high caloric intake, and use nutritive supplements. With AIDS, cryptosporidiosis may become chronic, and an individual may be subject to some periods of partial relief, followed by the return of severe symptoms.

Cytomegalovirus

Cytomegalovirus (CMV) is a common viral infection not associated solely with AIDS. CMV is a member of the herpes family of viruses, but distinct from the herpes simplex virus.

A large percentage of the population has had CMV infection at some time in their lives. There have been estimates compiled by the Centers for Disease Control and Prevention (CDC) that suggest that 90% of homosexual mean with HIV have been infected with CMV. CMV is usually asymptomatic and limited in those with a healthy immune system. A mildly symptomatic version is manifested by influenza-like symptoms: fever, aches, mild sore throat, weakness, and enlarged lymph glands.

A full-blown version of CMV causes encephalitis or ulcers in the colon or esophagus (gullet). If present in the liver, CMV can cause hepatitis; in the lungs, pneumonia; and in the eyes loss of vision, a condition called cytomegalovirus retinitis (CMVR). By itself, CMV causes at the least a mild form of immunosuppression and can reside in the body for up to 15 months before the infection is resolved. Of all described CMV developments, CMVR requires the most attention and is further discussed below.

CMV is transmitted via sweat, saliva, urine, or feces. It is also communicable in vaginal secretions and semen and is thus considered a sexually transmitted disease (STD) when appropriate. Severe CMV infection may be seen in terminal stages of AIDS. Although CMV infection can be controlled, there is no known cure.

CMV may be a co-factor in the development of full-blown AIDS. Diagnosis is readily made by taking a culture of body fluids.

Cytomegalovirus Retinitis

CMVR is an infection of the retina. Symptoms include sudden vision changes, increase in floaters (dark spots in the field of vision), and the distortion or absence of visual fields or areas. In addition, there may be a swelling of the retina that causes it to detach from the optic nerve.

CMVR is said to occur in 10% of all PWAs over time and is the most common CMVR symptom in those with AIDS. Loss of sight is possible if proper therapy is not applied in a timely manner. In fact, it is almost impossible to save the sight if CMVR enters the eye.

Case Study 1.3

Mark, a 40-year-old male, was admitted to the hospital with a high fever. Doctors suspected a CMV infection and drew blood to titer (a type of lab test that measures the amount of virus in a body). The test confirmed that there was indeed a CMV infection. Intravenous antibiotics were administered; however, Mark began to complain about a dullness of vision in his left eye. Over the next 2 weeks, his vision continued to worsen. By the time he was released, Mark had lost all vision in the eye, and his physician hoped to prevent it from crossing into the other eye.

Sudden or progressive worsening of CMV may be the result of another infection—either bacterial, fungal, or viral in nature. Therefore, CMVR may be much easier to treat if the other infection is treated along with it.

Enteropathy

Enteropathy is a noninfectious disease that typically features an inability of the GI tract to absorb nutrients and an impairment of gastric secretions.

Individuals with enteropathy are susceptible to enteric pathogenic agents, such as salmonella and helicobacteria, which can lead to chronic inflammation of the intestinal lamina propria (a subsurface layer of mucous membranes). Diagnosis of enteropathy is made by examining the blood for elevated mean corpuscular volume.

Esophagitis

Esophagitis is an inflammation of the esophagus and is often found in individuals with HIV. An early symptom may be pain in the upper or mid-chest. In addition, a regurgitation reflex may be seen.

It is most commonly caused by the organism *Candida*. Esophagitis is diagnosed by a barium swallow coupled with an endoscopic biopsy to determine whether its cause is viral or fungal (an endoscope is a thin, flexible instrument equipped with fiber optics and pincers for collecting tissue specimens).

Hairy Leukoplakia

Leukoplakia or oral leukoplakia is a fairly common viral infection that is sometimes mistaken for a form of fungus often called "thrush." Oral leukoplakia is thought to be caused at least in part by Epstein-Barr virus (EBV), which may be combined with human papillomavirus or HPV. It is distinguishable by white patches that appear on the sides of the tongue. Thicker than thrush, it cannot be scraped off without great difficulty.

Leukoplakia derives its name from the appearance of hairlike projections, similar to wet cotton or velvet. They may have a smooth, corrugated, or folded surface appearance.

In some people, leukoplakia may dissipate on its own, but in the presence of HIV, it is unlikely to do so. Symptoms of leukoplakia strongly indicate immune suppression.

Hepatitis

Hepatitis is characterized by an inflammation or infection of the liver. Depending on which type, hepatitis may be caused by a virus, microbes, toxic agents in the bloodstream, or immunological abnormalities.

Hepatitis A is transmitted by contaminated food or drink and is common where sanitation is poor. The carrier is a small RNA virus. After a 15- to 40-day incubation period, the affected person will develop a fever and feel ill. Approximately a week later, jaundice may develop and persist for as long as 3 weeks. Throughout this entire period, the infected person is contagious.

Serious physical complications seldom occur, and a childhood attack of hepatitis A (HA) is fairly common and often confers immunity.

Hepatitis B (serum hepatitis), or HBV, is transmitted by infected blood or needles contaminated with disease. HBV has on occasion been transmitted by tattooing with a contaminated needle. It is also considered a sexually transmitted disease when found to be caused by anal intercourse.

Long before the advent of AIDS, "Hep B" was known as a dangerous, sometimes deadly phenomenon within the groups first struck by HIV in the early 1980s. HBV is caused by a virus that can behave in many ways, including a chronic or acute state.

Symptoms may develop suddenly after an incubation period of 1–6 months and may include headache, fever, chills, weakness, and jaundice. GI distress is also likely, and can be accompanied by dark or discolored urine. Recovery is gradual for most. In the presence of HIV, HBV is much more likely to be serious or fatal.

There is a "Type C," often referred as "non-A, non-B" hepatitis, which is usually acquired through blood transfusions. It is caused by a virus related to the flavivirus. Type C has common hepatitis symptoms, but progression to a chronic condition may occur in up to 50% of those who contract it. Of these, perhaps 20% will suffer from cirrhosis. An exact diagnosis of this disorder is very difficult.

"Type D" or "delta" hepatitis seems to occur only with or after HBV infection. It is caused by a small, defective RNA virus and has grown to epidemic proportions in some locations. Hepatitis E is currently confined to third world countries. It is similar to hepatitis A. There is also a known autoimmune hepatitis that exists in several types referred to together as "lupoid." Lupoid hepatitis is characterized by an elevated immunoglobulin G (IgG) and antibody of what are called smooth-muscle types (antinuclear or antiactin). These disorders seem to affect women far more often than they do men.

Herpes Simplex Virus I

Herpes simplex virus I (HSV or HSV-1) is just one member of a family of viruses. HSV causes "cold sores" or "fever blisters" that appear on the lips and edges of the eyes and can also appear on the genitals.

Its counterpart, herpes simplex virus II (HSV-2), appears more often as sores on genital areas. Both strains are very common. Of the two, HSV-2 is more specifically spread by direct contact with other lesions. However, HSV can be transmitted without the presence of lesions. Like other herpes viruses, HSV-1 can lie dormant for random periods of time in lymphatic or nerve tissue before appearing and reappearing. In both HSV-1 and HSV-2, the presence of lesions occurs with an appearance of inflammation, tingling or itching, and then pain if pressure is applied to the mature and deep lesions.

Herpes and its typical symptomatic sores may spontaneously remit. They will also recur during illness and when the immune system is suppressed. At times, excessive exposure to sunlight or stress may bring on a bout of herpes. In rare cases, HSV appears about the ears or fingers and may be very painful.

HSV can be treated, but as with all viruses, there is no known cure. Diagnosis is made by obtaining a viral culture. People with compromised immune systems and individuals previously infected with the herpes virus can experience outbreaks of HSV that do not heal in the expected 7–14 days or that appear on other parts of the body such as the hands.

Herpes Simplex Virus II

Herpes simplex virus II (HSV II or HSV-2) is a virus that causes painful sores on the anus or genitals. Sexually transmitted, it is the second most common venereal disease or STD. When present in a PWA, the infection tends to persist and affect large areas. An infected mother may transfer this virus to her unborn child.

HSV II can be treated, but again, there is no known cure. HSV conditions lasting longer than 30 days in those with HIV can be considered a defined AIDS condition by the CDC.

Herpes Zoster

Herpes zoster (HZ), commonly called "shingles," is caused by the virus responsible for chicken pox and varicella-zoster. It affects the CNS, and after a few days of chills, fever, or GI problems, small raised lesions with inflamed bases may be evident. The lesions are tender and painful. After approximately 5 or 6 days, the patient will usually experience remission.

One attack of HZ leads to limited immunity against future outbreaks. Shingles, especially as seen in elderly persons, are temporary flare-ups of HZ.

In immunocompromised persons, as with PWAs, the involvement may persist and become more widespread. If lesions are still present after 10–14 days, the person may require antiviral treatment.

Histoplasmosis

Histoplasmosis is a fungal infection that often begins with flu- or pneumonialike symptoms. It is caused by the spores of *Histoplasma capsulatum*, which is often found in the midwestern United States, particularly in the Mississippi and Ohio River valleys. Symptoms can include a persistent cough, shortness of breath, fever, weakness, anemia, weight loss, and swollen glands. Histoplasmosis is rarely fatal but may become severe. It can cause inflammation of meninges, adrenal glands, heart, peritoneum, and other parts of the body. It can also cause acute pneumonia, a disease in which the lungs' ability to function is impaired because they become filled with fluid; this condition requires immediate attention.

Toxoplasmosis

Toxoplasmosis is usually preceded by latent *Toxoplasma* infection, although the latent form is fully active only in approximately 30% of PWAs.

To determine its presence, a positive test for *Toxoplasma gondii* antibody is performed. In addition, skin tests can identify persons with past exposure to histoplasmosis or coccidioidomycosis, two diseases with long, low-level dormant stages. Relapses of these diseases is uncertain, however; their appearance is just as likely to result from fresh exposure.

Candidiasis

Candidiasis is a fungal yeast infection usually caused by the organism *Candida albicans* and in rare cases by *Candida tropicalis*. *Candida* is considered part of the normal flora in certain parts of the body, such as the vagina or intestine.

During times of lowered immunity, *Candida* may spread to other parts of the body. It can cause recurrent vaginitis (vulvovaginal candidiasis, or yeast infections), which is a possible sign of HIV infection.

Candidiasis may cause jock itch or sinus infection. *Candida* infections may occur while taking an antibiotic because the antibiotic kills organisms that normally control *Candida* growth. Oral *Candida* infections are extremely common, especially in children. Commonly referred to as thrush, oropharyngeal candidiasis in the presence of HIV is a serious medical problem.

Candida symptoms include creamy patches of gray or white pus with the mucous membrane becoming inflamed and painful at the affected sites. Unlike a manifestation of hairy leukoplakia, this pus can be wiped or scraped off. This affliction is unsightly and worrisome to the affected person. Removal of this coating often exposes fiery red (erythematous) lesions.

The *Candida* infection may cover only part of the tongue or the entire inside of mouth. Although thrush is generally found on buccal mucosa, the palate, or the dorsum of the tongue, lesions may appear at several sites. Persons affected with thrush may experience a sore throat and a change in taste.

If thrush spreads to the esophagus, swallowing may become difficult. In addition, the respiratory tract may be affected. If the infection progresses from the mouth to the bronchi, trachea, or lungs, the diagnosis is "full-blown" AIDS.

Thrush may occur systemically and even affect the heart and the meninges. The *Candida* infection can also be found in the nailbeds, in the umbilicus (navel), and around the anus.

Candidiasis is diagnosed through a culture or a visual inspection of affected areas.

AIDS Dementia

AIDS dementia is one of the most common AIDS-related CNS pathologies. This syndrome may be due to the direct attack of HIV on the brain. The syndrome, also referred to as *HIV dementia* or *AIDS–dementia complex* (ADC), is estimated to occur in from 10% to 45% of individuals afflicted with AIDS, particularly in the end stages of AIDS.

Early symptoms may include mild forgetfulness, loss of concentration, and confusion. Motor-related symptoms may include loss of balance or leg weakness. Additional mental symptoms can follow, such as apathy, social withdrawal, and depression. Anxiety, with or without concurrent hypochondria, is also seen in AIDS dementia patients.

Over time, AIDS dementia can cause some memory loss, impaired thinking, loss of the ability to perform complex tasks, difficulty walking, and a greater loss of coordination. In highly developed AIDS dementia, the afflicted person will be bedridden and possibly incontinent. May AIDS dementia symptoms bear some resemblance to those of Alzheimer's disease.

It has been strongly recommended that when dementia is

suspected, the person be given proper neuropsychiatric testing and a complete examination including the nervous system.

There is no specific test for this illness. Therefore, other causes and illnesses that might imitate dementia must be ruled out as part of the diagnostic process.

Summary

AIDS is caused by a retrovirus named human immunodeficiency virus (HIV). The diagnosis of AIDS is made when a person is known to be infected with HIV and has either the presence of an opportunistic disease or a T-cell count below $200/mm^3$ of blood.

There are four steps that must occur for an HIV infection to establish itself:

1. The virus must become attached to a cell. HIV does this by recognizing the CD4 protein receptor site on the lymphocyte.
2. The virus must penetrate the cell to which it has attached itself.
3. The virus, once in the cell, implants its genetic code into the cell's genome. Thus, whenever the cell divides, it passes the virus' ability to reproduce on to the daughter cells.
4. The virus must replicate. This is done using the cell's metabolic machinery to reproduce the virus. Often in the process, the cell is destroyed.

Once HIV has taken over the immune system, there are indicators that this system is impaired. The body falls prey to diseases that will eventually kill the patient if the disease is not treated aggressively. Diseases that are lethal to the person who has AIDS are most often harmless to those who do not. Eventually, available treatments are unable to stop the many diseases that will continue to plague the individual.

The common symptoms of AIDS (not HIV infection) include sudden loss of 10 or more pounds in less than a month when not trying to diet; persistent coughs, colds, and flus; chronic diarrhea; bed-soaking night sweats; and chronic fatigue.

2

HIV Transmission
An Explanation of How HIV Moves from Person to Person

HIV is spread from person to person in ways that have become well known. It is mandatory that those who work in prevention, education, and treatment understand the methods of transmission. With this information, they can educate people to make changes in their behavior that can protect them from infection.

What modes of behavior are significant to HIV transmission? Who should take precautions and what precautions should be taken? When should these precautions be taken?

There must be three aspects of transmission in order for the virus to infect a person: (1) a point of exit from the infected individual, (2) a mechanism to transport the virus to another person, and (3) a point of entry into a second body. These aspects exist in the human dynamic every day. Sexual intercourse, injection drug use, and medicine each facilitate the virus's ability to spread from one person to another.

Sexual Intercourse and HIV Transmission

HIV is most frequently spread from one person to another during sex. In the United States, HIV has been seen most often in bisexual and homosexual males. This predominance is attributable to the nature of gay male sex, to gender, and to the size of the gay population.

The Gay Male Population

The gay male population in large metropolitan cities such as New York, San Francisco, and Miami was ideal for HIV infiltration. In these large cities, there were clubs, bathhouses, and bars that welcomed young gay men from all areas to come and be readily accepted by their peers. This environment gave gay men the opportunity to meet other gay men and form a social and sexual network; that is, these groups, like their heterosexual counterparts, made it easier to meet people, date, and possibly have intercourse. An important and often overlooked aspect of the seeming frequency of HIV transmission in this social order is not the sexual behaviors but the relatively small size of the gay male population. To fully understand this concept, it is important to know the difference between incidence and prevalence. *Incidence* is the rate at which a certain event occurs, that is, the number of new cases of a disease that occur during a specific period of time. *Prevalence*, by contrast, is the total number of cases in a given population at a given period of time.

Gay men represent somewhere between 3% and 10% of the population (depending on the source of the estimate). If this is the true percentage, it can be assumed that a city with a population of 100,000 people potentially has 10,000 gay citizens. Now take away 52% of this number to account for lesbians. This leaves 4800 gay men in the city. HIV, if introduced into this small population, would instantly have a high prevalence. Because of this high prevalence, there is more risk associated with gay sex. This can be a difficult concept to understand. How can HIV be more deadly in the gay population? Why would it not have been just as deadly in the heterosexual population? This is the wrong approach to understanding why the population had something to do with the rapid spread of HIV in the United States. There is an explanation: For example, imagine that there are two populations of people. One population numbers 100, and the other numbers 10. Both populations have a 10% HIV infection prevalence. Which population poses a greater risk of infection, the smaller one or the larger one? They are pretty much the same statistically, but there are two other aspects of this puzzle to look at when considering the gay male population as a co-factor for risk. The first is that human behavior is not always as random or as independent as a roll of dice. For instance, if one man were sleeping with two men concurrently, this would alter the statistics. If one man in each group has an affair, the percentage change is higher in the smaller population (20% in the smaller percentage, 12% in the larger). Couple this with the fact that most adults do have more than one sexual partner. This means that the percentage change continues to rise in the smaller population at a much higher rate. Which population would pose a greater threat to a newcomer? The answer is the smaller one. This is proven by the 8% difference in population prevalence seen in the example.

A smaller population is more dangerous with regard to transmission by virtue of the prevalence of HIV. When evaluating safe sex programs and prevention education, explaining this risk factor is particularly important. A young gay male faces more risk for HIV infection than does his heterosexual counterpart. Another aspect of transmission in gay males is the nature of gay sex compared to heterosexual sex. It is clear that the insertive partner, defined as the one who penetrates with his penis, in either heterosexual or homosexual intercourse faces less risk than the receptive partner. It is logical to assume that an individual who can be both insertive and receptive during sexual intercourse has a better chance not only of being infected, but also of transmitting the virus to another person. For instance, a man who has tested positive for HIV can transmit the virus to either a man or a woman. In contrast, a woman cannot be the insertive partner. Added to this greater risk posed by the male is the higher incidence of anal intercourse in the gay male population.

Anal Sex

The anus is not physiologically suited to intercourse. The tissues in this area of the body are delicate and tear easily when penetrated by a penis. The vagina, by comparison, is lubricated by mucous membranes and is more elastic and muscular. The act of anal intercourse often causes small tears that are susceptible to the HIV in the semen. Furthermore, HIV has a higher concentration in semen than in vaginal secretions. The semen contains the sperm, which the body protects with white blood cells as a function of insuring survival of the species.

In summary, the concentration of HIV in the gay male population is caused by the following factors: the population size, the ability to be both a receptive and an insertive sexual partner, the fact that semen has a higher concentration of HIV than vaginal fluids, and the practice of anal sex.

The greatest risk behavior for transmission of HIV is receptive anal intercourse without a condom. While much has been broadcast about the need for protected sex, there are still thousands of people having unprotected intercourse. Once it seemed that prevention education directed toward changing the sexual practices of gay men worked. Now it seems that more and more young gay males are infected. The following case study of a 25-year-old man named Brian illustrates the findings of recent studies:

Case Study 2.1

Brian is an attorney who lives in New York City and works in a small law firm. He had moved to New York to attend law school, but admitted that he also wanted to come to the city to experience being gay in a place where he would not be viewed as strange or perverted.

After law school, during a difficult period of failing and having to retake the bar exam, he went out and got drunk on more than one occasion and had sex with a few men whom he did not know. He did not use a condom during these nights with other men. He believes that this is when he was infected with HIV.

"I just never thought that I would get it, but I knew it was stupid," he explained. "I mean, I knew I could get HIV, I just thought I wouldn't. I guess another part of me also wanted to have sex with someone. I wanted these men at the time, and I guess I always thought there was a chance that one of these tricks might be a guy that I could really enjoy and fall in love with. Whatever it was at the time, I ultimately thought it would not happen to me. I guess I thought being gay was a lot like being a man. My brother goes out and gets laid by ten different women in a year, and I had sex three times and got HIV. I guess I thought that I was too young to die and I was not going to get HIV because I've only slept with five people in my whole life."

The prevalence of HIV is higher in gay men than in heterosexuals. This makes receptive anal intercourse more of a risk for gay men than for women. This does not mean that the possibility for transmission is not equal. Anal sex, for both men and women, is a risk. However, the higher prevalence of HIV in gay males makes it statistically more likely that a gay male will be infected compared to a woman also engaging in receptive anal sex.

Oral Sex

Performing oral sex is a risk behavior, though it is not thought to carry the same degree of risk as anal or vaginal intercourse, because tissues in the mouth are not as easily compromised. The risks are higher for a person performing the act on a male, since the penis is inserted into the mouth, and there is a high concentration of HIV in semen.

HIV transmission during oral sex is possible because there are often small nicks and cuts in the mouth. These cuts can go unnoticed, providing a possible route of transmission. Swallowing semen and vaginal fluids increases the chances of infection. More points of entry will most likely be exposed to the virus as it travels through the body. Furthermore, HIV can be absorbed through mucous membranes and cause infection.

Vaginal Sex

Vaginal intercourse without a condom is dangerous. Sex commonly causes small tears in the walls of the vagina. The vagina is also lined with mucous membranes that allow HIV to enter the bloodstream.

For males, the threat is less but not nonexistent. Unprotected vaginal sex poses a risk of HIV infection for men for the same reasons that it does for women. The urethra, like the vagina, is lined with a mucous membrane. HIV in vaginal secretions poses the same threat to these membranes as the secretions come into contact with this mucous membrane.

Kissing

It is a widely accepted theory that saliva does not contain a viral load substantial enough to cause an HIV infection. The viral load refers to the amount of virus that is found in a given amount of fluid. It is thought that it takes a high viral load to transmit. This means that the saliva has far too little virus to infect another person, but this fact does not negate the other risk that might be present when kissing. The blood from a cut or blister (for instance, herpes in the oral area, commonly called "fever blisters," is a common malady) can be a risk factor. However, casual kissing is most likely not very dangerous, as long as there are no cuts, blisters, or open sores.

The concept of ranking sexual behaviors as high, medium, or low risk is an odd concept from a prevention perspective. The following case exemplifies how people approach the idea of degrees of risk and how this thought paradigm might not be the most prudent approach to prevent transmission:

Case Study 2.2

As a prevention educator in the area of sexual assault, I teach young people healthy ways to relate to one another. This includes giving children information about sexual assault as well as sex education. Often the students ask me questions about AIDS and HIV. I also teach the HIV module of the required New York State Department of Health's Rape Crisis Counselor's Training Program to counselor trainees.

The question about what constitutes high and low risk comes up often in my training, and I explain that it is really a silly concept. It really does not matter how you get it, it is *if* you get it. However, with young people it is often harder to get the point across. Once I was talking to a group of 10th graders. A young man asked me what were the worst behaviors and what were the best behaviors. I told him that they were all risk behaviors and told him what I tell the adults I talk to when providing DOH training. The explanation was not working. So I asked him the following:

"It's like this: You are a guy facing north on a long, straight road. The sun is at 12 o'clock and you are deaf. Cars come speeding from the south in the right-hand lane at the rate of 1 an hour. In the left-hand lane, trucks come up the road at a rate of 15 per hour. There are no indicators warning you of approaching cars. What lane would you pick?" I asked the young man.

"The right one," he said confidently.

"Why not get out of the road?" I asked.

Injection Drug Use

The second most common cause of HIV transmission, next to sexual transmission, is the shared use of injection drug paraphernalia (colloquially called "works"). Such sharing is a risk factor only when a syringe or works are shared with a person who has HIV.

A syringe is composed of a needle, a cylinder, and a plunger. All parts of the syringe can contribute to the transmission of HIV from one person to another. The needle itself is an excellent instrument for introducing substances into the body and removing them. Other parts of the syringe are also factors of HIV transmission. Often the user will "boot," that is, insert a needle into a vein, then pull back on the plunger, and thereby draw blood into the syringe. This practice exposes the entire syringe to HIV. The individual who uses the needle next now has a fully contaminated instrument that will be in direct contact with the blood.

Many people have a difficult time understanding how the paraphernalia can transmit HIV from one person to another. To understand this concept, it is helpful to first understand how injection drugs are bought, prepared, and used.

The most common illicit drugs administered directly into a vein are heroin, cocaine, and steroids. Using these drugs in any form is illegal. Moreover, buying syringes requires a physician's prescription, which makes them very difficult to procure. Restrictions placed on the distribution of needles often cause sharing.

Since the drugs are sold illegally, the method used to package and transport them must be easy and convenient for rapid distribution. The preferred way of selling the drugs is in small envelopes in the form of "rocks" or powder.

The high from injecting drugs is more powerful than the high from inhaling them. This means that in order to achieve the most intense high, the user must change the drug from powder to liquid form by mixing the powdered drug with water and then heating the mixture over a flame. This is often done with a spoon over a candle. The heat causes the drug to dissolve in the water. The user can then draw the solution into the syringe and inject it.

Because these drugs are prepared without the benefit of quality control, they often contain contaminants. After the drug is "cooled," inert particles often are found in the liquid form and must be filtered from the liquid before injection is possible. Filtering is done by drawing the liquid through cotton. The user places a small amount of cotton between the needle and the reservoir, pulling the drug through the cotton, which traps the particles. The needle has been exposed to HIV and is able to transmit it to another user.

Another aspect of paraphernalia acting as a mechanism for transmission is the use of a water glass to rinse the needle. When the liquid drug begins to cool, it crystallizes and clogs the needle. To remedy this problem, the needle is filled from and plunged into a glass of water. Like the cotton, the water glass acts as a reservoir for HIV, just waiting for the next user to rinse the needle.

Tissue Transplants and Blood Transfusions

In the beginning of the AIDS epidemic in the United States, HIV transmission from transplants and transfusions was much more common than it is today. At that time, there was no way to ascertain which blood or organ transplant donors were carrying the virus that caused AIDS because the causative agent had not been identified. Once AIDS was known to be a disease transmitted from person to person, there were efforts to screen out donors who fit the profile of a carrier. This screening translated into discouraging gay men from donating blood.

In 1986, the ability to screen blood and tissue donations for the presence of the HIV antibody dramatically reduced the incidence of HIV transmission from transplants and transfusions. Currently, because of unreliable testing techniques (which are more fully explored in Chapter 4), there are cases of infection due to transplants, but they are rare compared to what they once were. On the other hand, there are more cases of HIV transmission from these procedures today (according to the CDC, approximately 2000 people will be infected this year from transplants and transfusions) than the total number of AIDS cases recorded in 1982.

Occupational Exposures

Nurses, doctors, lab technicians, and others who work with sharp objects and HIV-positive people have been infected in the workplace. The most common cause of infections is an accidental needle stick. There have been reports of people being infected after being exposed to a blood spill, but these cases are extremely rare, as blood spills are very ineffective mechanisms for transmission. When blood is spilled, it often comes into contact with many things that destroy HIV, such as bleach and other cleaners. Furthermore, HIV needs to gain access to the bloodstream, and with the many layers of clothes that people wear, as well as other protective barriers, access to the bloodstream is very difficult.

Transmission from Mother to Child

A much-talked about method of HIV transmission is that which takes place between mother and child. Such transmission may occur in one of three ways: absorption of HIV crossing the placenta through the mucous membranes of the fetus, exposure to the mother's blood during the birth process, or ingestion of breast milk. (The issues that surround HIV transmission from mother to child are fully discussed in Chapter 7.)

Summary

HIV is a virus that must find its way into the bloodstream of an individual in order for infection to occur. This can happen in a variety of ways, all of them well documented. For prevention purposes, it is important that educators understand the ways that transmission can occur and be able to identify the three components of transmission that must occur in order for transmission to take place:

Point of exit: The point of exit refers to how HIV leaves the infected individual and infects another person. Sexual intercourse is the most frequent mode of HIV transmission. The points of exit for HIV during sexual intercourse are the penis and vagina. Occasionally, depending on the individual, the point of exit might be an open sore (for example, in a person with herpes).

For women who give birth to an HIV-positive child, the point of entry might have been the placenta or the tears in the vaginal walls during childbirth. For children infected after birth, the point of exit is the breast. This infection takes place during breast feeding.

Mechanism of transport: The mechanism of transport refers to the medium that carries HIV from the point of exit to the point of entry into another being. This can be blood, semen, breast milk, vaginal fluids, organs, or blood products used in medical procedures.

Point of entry: The point of entry refers to the location at which HIV enters another human being. This would be the mucous membranes of the rectum, mouth, vagina, and penis, as well as openings in the skin such as cuts, open sores, and abrasions.

Infection sites would be the point of entry for injection drug users and others who become infected during occupational exposures.

For children who become infected through the ingestion of breast milk, the points of entry are sores in the mouth, or the mucous membranes of the digestive tract, or both.

3

The History of AIDS and the Human Immunodeficiency Virus

Many books, including this one, refer to the year 1981 as the start of the AIDS epidemic, but that is not when HIV came into being. It was the time at which AIDS began to be recognized as a discrete disease. The year 1981 was identified retrospectively at the beginning of the AIDS epidemic. In 1981, doctors were aware only that they were seeing something unusual, in that young men were coming down with rare diseases. In March 1981, there were a few cases of a rare cancer called Kaposi's sarcoma. Few people at the time knew about this cancer, and those who were aware of it were surprised to see it in these young gay men, as they did not fit the profile for the usual Kaposi's sarcoma patient.

Kaposi's sarcoma (KS) was first identified in 1872 by Austrian dermatologist Moritz Kaposi, who named the cancer *sarcoma idiopathicum multiplex hemorrhagicum*. He described a slowly progressing disease with physical symptoms of purple nodules that appeared on the lower extremities and connective tissues. The men who were seen by Dr. Kaposi (there were three) all died within 3 years of their diagnosis.

In March 1981, several young men were identified as having lesions that were similar to KS. However, these men were younger and their ethnic heritage did not seem to be a factor. Their symptoms were unlike those of the classic form of KS (the form identified by Dr. Kaposi), in which the nodules appeared mostly on the extremities and connective tissues with accompanying symptoms of general swelling of lymph nodes. In these cases, the nodules appeared on the trunk and the face. The patients also had weight loss, fatigue, and a loss of appetite.

The fact that many of these men were young, and otherwise healthy, was another cause of concern. Men this age were not supposed to get this disease! Some doctors, upon hearing of these cases, came forward and said that they had seen KS in some of their patients who had immune system disorders.

In the late 1970s and early 1980s, major milestones were reached in the transplantation of organs and tissues as a result of immunosuppressive medications. In order to successfully transplant a foreign tissue into the body of another person, the recipient's immune system must be suppressed enough to enable the new tissues to exist without being attacked by the host's immune system. The introduction of drugs such as cyclosporine made transplants more viable, and thus more common. Other immune-suppression therapies for diseases such as lupus also created a population of people who were immune-suppressed. These were people who, due to another etiology, were on occasion presenting to doctors with symptoms of KS that were atypical as well. These cases of KS were attributed to either the lack or the impairment of the immune system. It was the effect on this population, those whose immune systems were deliberately suppressed, that gave doctors and epidemiologists the first clue that the cancers being observed in this population were indicators that immune dysfunction was occurring.

There were also cases of Pneumocystis carinii pneumonia being documented at the New York Hospital Cornell University School of Medicine in people who were not historically at risk for this disease. Pneumocystis carinii pneumonia (PCP), like KS, was an infection that was not seen in people whose immune systems were functioning. When seen in people who were not medically immunosuppressed, these diseases (referred to as *opportunistic infections*) were reported to the Centers for Disease Control (CDC; since redesignated the Centers for Disease Control and Prevention). The one significant clue to this unfolding mystery was that all the people who were identified as having either KS or PCP were homosexual men. In 1981, there were 42 cases of either KS or PCP reported to the CDC. In 1982, the number had jumped to 340. By the end of that year, the number of cases had reached over 1000. It was at this point that an "epidemic" was recognized by the CDC, though there was still no identifiable source (etiology) of the disease or any risk factors that could be identified. All that was known at this point was that there was something deadly affecting gay men under 40 years of age. It appeared to be transmitted, but how and when transmission took place was unknown. What could be inferred from the incidence of the disease from January 1981 to January 1983 was that the disease seemed to be transmitted from person to person. The one clue that epidemiologists had was that this disease seemed to be affecting gay men in certain cities. What this suggested was open to interpretation.

Gay-Related Immunodeficiency

There has been a lot of clamoring, by groups such as the AIDS Coalition to Unleash Power (ACT UP), a New York City–based grassroots organization, that public health officials were too slow in identifying AIDS as a threat to the public's health. Realistically, though, the first few cases did not yield enough information to state definitely that there was something going on in any particular population. The numbers of people who had these rare diseases were minuscule compared to the general population. Because homosexuals were the only people identified as entering this "disease population" at the time, research made homosexuality a criterion for identification. Researchers started to record the numbers of gay men who were diagnosed with immune system disorders and correctly postulated that the disease was acquired. Using these pieces of information, the infection of gay men, the immune system failing, and the theory that the disease was acquired, they coined the designation GRID (for gay-related immunodeficiency). In March 1981, the CDC released two reports, one on Kaposi's sarcoma and the other on Pneumocystis carinii pneumonia occurring in homosexual men. Medical professionals who saw gay men with opportunistic infections were encouraged to report them to local health departments. In July 1981, there were only 41 cases of this phenomenon nationwide—hardly enough cases to sound the alarm about a dangerous epidemic. There were still no clues about the cause of GRID. Researchers thought it might have stemmed from drug use or from an unknown physiological difference between homosexual and heterosexual people.

Gay life in the early 1980s was largely a mystery to the population as a whole. The fact that some homosexuals frequented bathhouses and sex clubs was not generally known to health officials or to the general public outside of large cities. The CDC had conducted studies that investigated the transmission of hepatitis in gay men, and these studies suggested that the transmission rate was higher in the homosexual population, attributed to the nature of some gay sex (anal intercourse). GRID was not initially identified as a communicable disease with the potential of infection because of the lack of information about the etiology of the disease. What was known in 1981 was that there was a disease that was affecting young gay men in major cities. They came to hospitals and doctors' offices with rare cancers and opportunistic infections. Their immune systems seemed to be under some sort of attack, but the source of and reason for this attack were still a mystery.

It had not been shown that gay men were exclusively susceptible to GRID, but the link between homosexuality and GRID was apparent because all the people who had the problem with their immune systems were gay. The researchers (epidemiologists, physicians, and public health officials) therefore started to examine the differences between gay and straight lifestyles.

The obvious difference between gay and heterosexual men was that the former group was more likely to be sexually exposed to other men's semen. The question became whether the introduction of semen into the bloodstream could weaken the immune system to such a point that infections of this sort could take hold. While there was some information that large doses of foreign tissue could tax an immune system, it seemed rather unlikely that this was actually happening in the case of GRID. Homosexuality, anal intercourse, and other variants of human sexuality were not new. If they were the cause, there surely would have been some sort of prior history of the disease.

Another aspect of gay life in the early 1980s was the use of nitrate inhalants known as "poppers." They were sold in liquid form and gave off a vapor that was in turn inhaled by the user to achieve a state of euphoria. These drugs, used almost exclusively by gay men, were extremely popular. It was thought that nitrate inhalants could suppress the immune system of some, but not all, individuals, and that they could affect a small number of people within the gay community. Now this theory is rejected. At the time, there was not enough information about the disease itself to exclude nitrate inhalants as reasonable causative agents. They were seen as such because there are certain chemical compounds, such as benzene, that can cause certain cancers. Researchers had little information about the effects of nitrate inhalants on the immune system.

In 1982, according to the CDC, there were 340 cases of GRID, almost all of which involved homosexual men in major cities in the United States. It was clear that there was something very different occurring in this population. It was known that there was a higher incidence of certain sexually transmitted diseases in gay male populations. Hepatitis, for example, was known to be a blood-borne pathogen that disproportionally affected gay men. But it was yet to be determined that GRID was a disease that was blood-borne or transmitted sexually.

It was during this time (1982) that Dr. Robert Gallo, a researcher at the National Cancer Institute, isolated and identified the first retrovirus, named HTLV (human thymocyte leukemia virus). This virus was thought to cause a rare form of leukemia. The significance of this discovery was that the virus attacked the leukocyte, the immune system cell charged with protecting the body from harm.

While Dr. Gallo was in the process of discovering the retrovirus at the NCI, public health officials were conducting cluster studies to examine the relationship between individual GRID cases. For several reasons, it took time to establish a connection between cases. For one, the disease had a long period between infection and symptoms of full-blown GRID. At this time, it had not yet been discovered that the initial infection might resemble the flu. Because of the length of time between exposure and disease, it was hard to find out who had had sexual relations with whom. Furthermore, institutions such as bathhouses and sex clubs made casual and anonymous sex more available, contributing to the difficulty of conducting cluster studies.

In 1983, cases of GRID were discovered in heterosexual men. Most of these men were hemophiliacs—males born with a genetic metabolic error that precluded them from making factor VIII, the protein responsible for blood clotting. These young males were very prone to hemorrhaging. To combat the problems associated with the inability to clot, researchers developed a method to isolate factor VIII by pooling large quantities of blood from multiple donors. The result was the ability to deliver factor VIII alone to those who needed it and not make them suffer through large transfusions of blood. Unfortunately, it also exposed them to hundreds of people's blood every time they needed factor VIII.

As time passed, cases were discovered in other people who had received blood transfusions. The disease now seemed to be transmitted not only through sexual activity, but also through the use of blood products. It became apparent that this was a transmittable disease and was not caused by gay men or endemic only in that population. The name GRID was changed to AIDS after pressure from civil-rights-minded researchers who suggested that "GRID" caused a negative focus on the already-vilified homosexual and that it lent a false sense of security to people who were not homosexual but who were nonetheless at risk for the disease. On December 10, 1982, the CDC released a notice through one of its publications, the *Morbidity and Mortality Weekly Report* (*MMWR*), that this disease, now known as acquired immunodeficiency syndrome, might be transmitted from person to person through sexual contact, sharing needles with an infected person, and transfusion of blood products. The story was telecast on every major network news program.

Although it was clear that AIDS was a biological phenomenon not exclusive to the homosexual population, the fact that gay men had the highest incidence of infection fueled an already significant antigay sentiment. Fundamentalists and right-wing extremists, for example, perceived AIDS as a manifestation of God's abomination of homosexuality. If God was willing to inflict His wrath on gays, there was little reason to think that mere mortals would be obligated to be kind to them.

While the cause of the disease was still unknown, doctors and researchers grew confident that the disease was caused by a virus. Blood tests of those infected with AIDS showed an imbalance in certain specialized white blood cells, specifically the CD4 T helper lymphocyte. The attack on the white cell by this unknown pathogen was similar to that of the retrovirus HTLV, discovered by Dr. Gallo and thought to cause a rare form of leukemia.

Dr. Gallo and his associates suggested that HTLV might be the cause of AIDS. They isolated the HTLV virus in AIDS patients, but failed to isolate it in any other cases. Concurrently, Dr. Luc Montagnier, a leading French virologist at the Pasteur Institute in Paris, isolated yet another retrovirus thought to be responsible for AIDS.

The competition between the French and the Americans was heated, and by most accounts it was the French who first isolated a retrovirus common to all AIDS patients. The virus that causes AIDS was discovered as a result of a combined effort on the part of the French and Americans, through a jointly written series of papers. In 1986, it was announced that the cause of AIDS had been isolated and that there would soon be a test to detect its presence in the blood.

Researchers at the CDC, led by Dr. Donald Francis, were already aware that there was correlation between hepatitis and HIV. This was not a causal relationship, but there was a correlation: 80% of those with AIDS tested positive for hepatitis. While the hepatitis screening tests were not specific in weeding out or

identifying HIV, it was at the time the most accurate method to
remove infected blood from the blood supply. At this point, Dr.
Francis recommended that all blood banks test and subsequently
destroy all blood that tested positive for hepatitis. Officials from
the Red Cross and other blood banks thought Dr. Francis was an
alarmist and decided not to screen for hepatitis as a marker for
HIV. Later, blood-screening tests in San Francisco and other metropolitan areas showed that 1 in 500 people who received blood
transfusions contracted HIV.

The battle between the French and Americans was again
brewing, this time for the patent rights for an HIV screening test.
Dr. Gallo claimed credit for the discovery of HIV and felt that the
Americans deserved the patent rights. The French, in turn, thought
that the rights should be awarded to them.

While the scientific community was busy fighting over the
credit for discovering the cause of AIDS, the United States government was slow to address both the spread of HIV and the needs of
those who were already infected. There were officials who believed that HIV was a disease that would remain exclusive to gay
men and was not a problem in or for the heterosexual community.
For this reason, little was done in the area of prevention education
that was designed for heterosexual audiences. There was still fear
of and prejudice against those suffering from AIDS, but the government did nothing to address methods of protection from HIV
transmission or to provide information that would help to combat
fear and prejudice.

In sharp contrast to the federal government, certain local
governments were aggressive in their efforts to address the AIDS
crisis. The city of San Francisco's health department ordered all
bathhouses to be closed in 1985. Soon after, New York City did the
same. Some bathhouses served as many as 1000 gay male clients
per day; it was clear that this was a very large avenue for the
spread of HIV, and closing the institutions that facilitated transmission of HIV was a good thing. But many gay rights activists
interpreted this move as another attempt to push them back into
the closet. The attention attracted by the move was therefore both
positive and negative. Clearly, it was inappropriate for public

health officials to allow this type of behavior to continue unchecked; however, attention was now focused on gay men spreading HIV through behavior that was often viewed as immoral. Even those who accepted homosexuality as a facet of humanity, including many gay men, had problems endorsing these self-indulgent behaviors in the face of an epidemic.

AIDS was still a disease that was thought primarily to be a killer of gay men, even though officials now knew that HIV was increasingly infecting hemophiliacs, recipients of blood transfusions, and those who had used contaminated needles for the injection of illegal drugs.

In 1985, the world learned that film star Rock Hudson suffered from AIDS. He became the first public figure known to have AIDS, and the public's ability to ignore AIDS began to crumble. By this time, grassroots organizations already had formed to deal with the emerging AIDS crisis. In New York City, the Gay Men's Health Crisis (GMHC) was formed to assist those with AIDS and provide support to their loved ones. To help change government policy in all areas concerning AIDS, ACT UP was formed. ACT UP used civil disobedience to call attention to the Reagan administration's silence. Attention was drawn to the FDA's procedures that kept drugs in clinical trials for years and to the lack of resources that were allocated to help prevent the spread of HIV. Many activists felt that the long period of time required to run clinical tests on potential therapies was pointless because the risk of taking a poorly researched therapy still had better odds for a cure compared to no treatment.

It was not only gay-organized groups that identified President Ronald Reagan and his administration as being inadequate in their response to the AIDS crisis in the United States. The Institute of Medicine, a department of the National Academy of Sciences, charged that the administration's approach to the AIDS crisis was wholly inappropriate. This organization issued a report calling for federal funding to help educate the public on ways to prevent transmission. Ironically, at the same time, the federal government cut funding to the CDC's educational effort to stop further AIDS transmission because it was felt inappropriate to provide education on how to perform sodomy. This was not what the CDC was educating people about, of course, but the perception that it was, fostered by politicians such as Jesse Helms, was enough to cut the funding.

The president was now under enormous pressure from activists, the CDC, and other groups to acknowledge that AIDS did exist. Up to this point, Ronald Reagan had not publicly addressed the disease or those affected by it. The president's response to the AIDS epidemic was to ask the surgeon general for a report.

C. Everett Koop was a pediatrician who was appointed to the post of Surgeon General of the United States in 1981. He was, by all accounts, a conservative man with deep religious convictions. He was a leader in the field of pediatric surgery and was also a staunch opponent of abortion. In Washington circles, he was thought of as an eccentric. He wore a military uniform in keeping with the post of surgeon general. At the time of his appointment, gay rights leaders and proponents of women's issues opposed his nomination.

After spending a year reading reports and talking to people who were informed about the issues concerning AIDS and HIV, the surgeon general did something no one—not gay rights activists, not AIDS activists, not political commentators, not the president— had expected: Dr. Koop looked at the issues and wrote a report based on the public's interest in controlling the virus that was thought to cause AIDS. He recommended the use of condoms to prevent infections transmitted through sexual contact. He urged people to clean their "works" if they were insistent upon using drugs. The report called for frank education about sexuality and methods of preventing infection. It further rejected the ideas of mandatory testing and quarantine because the surgeon general thought that such actions would only further add to the stigma associated with HIV and AIDS. To the surgeon general, this was a dangerous dynamic.

His frank and open discussion of the issue was viewed as a complete divergence from the conservative party line. What many in the Reagan administration did not realize at the time was that C. Everett Koop was first and foremost a physician, not a politician. His medical background was a progressive one of pioneering surgeries and treatment for children, and his views on abortion were based not only on his theological principles but also on his medical training. He believed, for example, that the fetus, although dependent on the mother, was a separate being because the information that identifies an individual is its unique genome. The Reagan administration's flaw in evaluating Dr. Koop was that they thought him to be, based on his history of antiabortion activity, a person who would follow the party line.

The Reagan administration failed to realize that it was the very conviction that compelled Dr. Koop to advocate against abortion that would motivate him to take a liberal stance on a very hot issue. By understanding the need that society had for a realistic picture of those infected with the virus, and by developing a workable plan to reduce both the prevalence and the incidence of the disease, Dr. Koop offered a voice of authority. While some were saying that it was too little too late, it was nonetheless a start. The surgeon general's open support of gay-targeted educational plans, as well as frank discussion of other sensitive issues, such as how to clean needles to avoid spreading the virus, all furthered the respect for this man in those who once mercilessly slammed him. For the first time, there seemed to be a person with political power who acknowledged the plight of those infected with HIV with intelligence and insight.

In 1986, the federal government instituted a requirement that the blood bank industry test blood products for HIV infection. There were still those who thought such an act was extreme. After all, the number of people infected with AIDS was still small, and the number of those infected by tainted blood products was even smaller compared to the general population. The point lost was that a high proportion of people who received transfusions had a chance of becoming infected with HIV. The CDC estimated that over 80% of hemophiliacs were infected with HIV because they had received contaminated factor VIII blood.

It is constructive to look back at the way the epidemic was addressed and to find fault with the way officials handled the crisis, if there can be some type of value gained from such an analysis. It is important to explore the very factors that were often overlooked in the early evaluation of the AIDS crisis, because it was these very factors that made HIV more prevalent.

HIV, like hepatitis, is a blood-borne pathogen and is difficult to transmit from person to person. The ability of the virus to infect people, and thus its ability to spread, is determined by the behavior and size of the infected group. Unfortunately, politicians, religious leaders, civil rights activists, and the medical community all failed to explain in simple terms to the vast majority of people the factors that had caused the AIDS epidemic.

HIV has become prevalent because of changes that have occurred over the past few decades in the global community. HIV is not a new virus; it has existed for decades without having the effect on mankind that is seen today. In 1952, a doctor in Manchester, England, had a patient who died a mysterious death. He froze a specimen of this man's blood in hopes that one day future medicine would be able to see what this man suffered from. With the use of a complicated testing technique known as a polymerase chain-reaction test (PCR), it was confirmed that this man did in fact have AIDS. This suggested that HIV was not new, but that something changed in the environment, allowing HIV to enter into the population and find an active and efficient route of transmission.

HIV's natural reservoir, that is, where the virus is thought to reside or originate, is not known, but it is thought to be in Africa—the largest and most dynamic continent on the globe. The varied nature of the African continent provides insight into the origin of the AIDS epidemic. HIV and man have existed together for decades without the mass loss of life that is seen today. The reason is probably not that the virus has mutated and become more virulent and lethal, but more likely that it has been given access to more people. It may be that HIV, in its natural reservoir, posed little threat to the inhabitants of the area. It is also possible that HIV, in its natural reservoir, did not come into contact with man. Man has long been encroaching into areas that he had not previously inhabited. This penchant for exploring and conquering new territories might be part of the reason HIV is now prevalent. Human domi-

nation of the natural environment, with little regard for what
hazards might result, is well documented. The infiltration of a
migrating group into an indigenous population has often resulted
in the devastation of the latter. In the 1600s and 1700s, thousands of
Native American people were infected with influenza, causing
widespread deaths. The large-scale morbidity that was seen occurred because the flu was not something that the immune systems of Native Americans could fight. It is plausible that the
introduction of HIV to people who are not native to the natural
reservoir causes a similar reaction, and although this might explain why HIV causes such devastation, it does not explain the
rapid rate of infection across the globe.

Amplification of HIV in the United States

Changing societal norms and the introduction of certain tech-
nologies caused HIV to become so prevalent, but these phenom-
ena are not often covered in the press or by activists and educators
who try to educate people about HIV. This omission, an unfortu-
nate one, most likely comes about because these aspects are not as
interesting as sex and drug use. These are the things that sell, not
the long explanations that deny the ability to blame, ridicule, or
at best generate controversy; yet changes in technology and behavioral norms explain the prevalence of HIV without assigning
blame to any particular group. To understand the stunning effect
that technology has had on the ability of HIV to infect so many
people that it is now no longer endemic but rather pandemic, it is
important to look at some of the changes that occurred in the place
where HIV is though to originate—Africa.

The Colonization of Africa

Africa is a continent so dynamic that to live in one corner
demands skill and adaptation that might well preclude one from

living in another area. Those living in the deserts or savannas of Africa have developed certain adaptations that allow them to survive in the extreme heat with little water. Nomadic herding populations pass down from generation to generation information such as the locations of watering holes and routes to take during dry seasons, information that allows existence in a climate that seems from an outsider's view to be an uninhabitable environment. But adaptation to an environment does not stem only from learning. As science has begun to unravel the genetics of man, it has become clear that certain populations have genetic advantages that others do not.

In certain geographic areas, specifically those near riverbeds and marshes, malaria was endemic. It was discovered that people in these areas often carried the gene responsible for sickle cell anemia. When only one gene for sickle cell anemia is present (a status referred to a *heterozygous*), as opposed to both genes (*homozygous*), the person does not have the disease sickle cell anemia, but rather has the sickle cell trait. Genetic researchers discovered that in this environment, the sickle cell trait is actually advantageous because those with the trait are more resistant to malaria. It is no surprise that certain populations develop physiological adaptation to their environment; such adaptation is routinely seen in the animal world.

The difference in environment from one region to another, as well as a group's adaptation to its particular surroundings, collectively acted as a natural barrier against migration. Rivers were rarely crossed because of the dangers of hippo and crocodile attacks. The change of environment from grasslands to rainforests reduced the chance of migration. One group possessed traits that would give them advantages on flat, uncluttered areas. Height gave an advantage to nomadic herding people because it allowed them to see farther and use that advantage to avoid predators of their livestock. Those living in the rainforest tended to be shorter, making it easier to navigate through thick, low-hanging vegetation. It is seen throughout the races that certain traits support living in certain environments. Inuit Indians, who inhabit the Arctic region, can fish in icy waters and not suffer frostbite when they use their bare hands to perform these tasks; they have developed a circulatory system with a superior ability to warm their hands and feet.

As Africa was colonized by Europeans, natural boundaries were changed, and so were the lifestyles of the native people. Boundaries that had been established by nature were now being redesigned by men who had little knowledge of what the consequences might be. Construction of roads greatly accelerated travel. It became possible to reach isolated areas and cultures quickly and often. The resulting invasion meant that people who had never been exposed to certain environments were now being exposed to foreigners bringing foreign diseases. The continent was now changing from independent groups of people into a pluralistic community. The repercussions of this new pluralism meant that agents that were native and harmless to one population would now enter new areas and cause harm to indigenous populations. There was sharing not only of technology and culture, but also of disease. The effort to conquer the "Dark Continent" was not motivated solely by politics. Religious colonizations often took the form of missionary work, which included the introduction of Western medical services. Vaccination, for example against childhood diseases, commenced on a large scale.

The process of urbanization concentrated people in newly formed cities where sanitation was often substandard. The enormous need for medical attention to combat the health problems of urban poverty was daunting. Confronted with a lack of supplies, medical workers often solved the lack by re-using hypodermic syringes. Thus, diseases that were difficult to transmit through casual contact found a more certain means of transmission.

Along with the pluralization of African cultures and the development of political borders came a dilution of values that were connected to heritage. Now, marriages between tribes could take place, when once they were unheard of if for no other reason than that the environment was too restrictive to provide an opportunity to meet others (except in cases of tribal warfare).

Additionally, the introduction of Western diseases such as syphilis and herpes became a factor in HIV transmission in this area. Many of the diseases that Europeans suffered from were not seen in native populations. Their bodies had no defense against these diseases, the symptoms of which included genital sores. With open sores on the genitals, sexual relations became extraordinarily dangerous if a person had HIV. These sores allowed for transmission of blood-borne pathogens between people at a much greater rate.

These changes explain how HIV gained a foothold in Africa. The next question is how the virus entered the Western world. The invention of air travel allowed a person to leave Africa and return in a matter of days. The development of social networks that encouraged people to explore the world for opportunity, as well as immigration policies and visa programs, provided the virus a transport mechanism to the United States and other nations. Still, this was not enough to cause an epidemic. The modern AIDS epidemic in the United States was caused by a host of technological advances and changes in behaviors that were not seen before the 1960s. These social changes, coupled with scientific advancements, made individuals from different societies more intimate with one another.

The Sexual Revolution

The sexual revolution of the 1960s and 1970s was a movement that had not been seen before in modern times. The idea that sex should be an act that was restricted to marriage was questioned and considered to be antiquated. "Free love" and sexual experimentation with multiple partners became acceptable and chic. This changing norm acted as an amplifier for many sexually transmitted diseases (STDs). The incidence of herpes, chlamydia, and other venereal diseases rose dramatically during this period. While these diseases had long been recognized, the ability to cure them was relatively new. At the turn of the century, many of these diseases were treated with sulfa drugs that did not always work; it was the introduction of antibiotics that provided health care workers with new and effective methods of treating these diseases. The available treatments lessened the threat that STDs once carried. One barrier against STDs, the fear of their deadliness, had been destroyed, and people felt less compelled to be careful in their choice of sex partners. ✓

The sexual revolution was not restricted to the heterosexual population. Homosexuals were engaged in their own sexual revolution. Identifying themselves as individuals who were interested in people of the same sex was only one part of the sexual revolution for gays and lesbians. Commercialized sex in the newly formed gay community became a popular institution in the gay male population. Bathhouses, for example, were opened in large cities across the nation following the gay sexual revolution (see Chapter 8, "Gay Men").

Case Study 3.1

Scott, a 42-year-old gay male, was diagnosed with AIDS in 1988. He had spent a great deal of time in the bathhouses in New York City and believes that he was infected with HIV from this activity. He has lost 32 pounds, has KS, and has already been treated for oral thrush, Pneumocystis carinii pneumonia, and a host of other opportunistic infections. He is one of the few men I have spoken to who will discuss his experience in the bathhouses:

"I was in college in New Paltz, and would go down to the city a lot. There were a lot of gays on campus, but I was not openly gay. I heard about the bathhouses when I was at a party. I thought that the people must have been kidding. I was curious because I thought it might be a good way to be with a man without people finding out. I was still so against being gay, I told people that I was straight. I dated women. I was so into being heterosexual I thought that this was the only place that I could go to explore my sexuality. I never really thought about all the other stuff that goes along with sex, such as love and intimacy. These were still things that I was not willing to identify as part of being a gay person. I went to the city one Saturday and went to the Village. I asked a person who I thought was gay about the baths, and he told me where to go.

"When I got into the bathhouse, it was like nothing I had ever seen before. The men were all so good-looking. They were all over the place. The attendant gave me a key to a room and a pile of towels. The room had a cot in it, and I remember to this day the smell of chlorine, sex, and smoke. I sat on the cot, and about five minutes later a guy shows up in the doorway and starts talking to me. I had oral sex with him. I felt really guilty about this when I got back to campus, but it was also like I had found something that I was looking for all my life. I started going back once a month or so, and I would have sex with a couple of guys each visit. I would go on a Sunday afternoon and spend about five hours having sex with a bunch of different men. I had thoughts that what I was doing might not be the smartest thing in the world, but I never thought that I would be getting sick. Even before HIV was talked about, I was getting sick. I had herpes, chlamydia, and gonorrhea. In 1981, I started to feel really bad, and I was diagnosed with hepatitis. I kind of knew that I was at risk for AIDS when it was first thought to be transmitted sexually. I figure that I slept with over 400 men at the baths. I was a kid, and I don't think that any kid, gay or straight, would turn down a place where all your peers are beautiful and available. It was a sexual playground. I look back now and I think, God what an unhealthy practice, even if there were no HIV, it's just not good for the mind and stuff. They were really unreal, it was just hundreds of men having sex all over the place."

The bathhouses that commercialized gay male sex also became a symbol of gay rights. The sex was not looked at as deviant behavior, but as an accepted part of the social tapestry. With no social taboos discouraging anonymous sex, the gay community was already at risk for an epidemic of sexually transmitted diseases.

Social conventions also put this population at risk. Without the possibility of a marriage contract, which at least suggests if it does not actually require monogamy, and with a social system that offered no support to same-sex relationships (health education targeted at gay males and their health issues was rarely available), a sexually transmitted, terminal disease introduced to this population was devastating. Not unlike the gay male population, another group that was considered "fringe" in that they were not conventional were the young people who were growing up and experimenting with drugs—drugs that people easily became addicted to.

The Drug Culture

During the 1960s, a significant movement against conventional thinking was formed, largely brought about by the Vietnam War. At 18 years of age, young men and women were being shipped off to foreign lands to fight for a cause that many of them did not understand. The legal voting age, however, was 21, and many of those going to war were not yet this age. The inability to vote, coupled with the reality of having to fight for a governmental goal not well understood, provoked many young people to protest. They rejected not just the Vietnam War, but the institutions that supported it. Groups such as the Black Panthers and the Weathermen sprang up. The climate was hostile; there were racial problems, protests against the war, and a division between the young and the old. Rejecting the societal norms of the time became a revolution of the younger generation. No longer did they heed words that warned against drug use and promiscuous sex. The younger generation accepted behaviors that were once thought to be deviant. The drugs that were once thought to be dangerous and illicit were now in vogue.

Certainly drugs were used before the 1960s, but those that had previously been taken were very different from those that have since become popular. Chemical advances allowed for the production of more concentrated substances such as LSD. Test tubes, burners, and chemical compounds that were needed to process substances into powerful drugs were available to all those who were interested in obtaining them. Not only were there more drugs, but also using them could and did cause addiction.

The administration of these drugs was also different. The development of plastics allowed for the inexpensive mass manufacturing of hypodermic needles. With this new method of administering drugs, HIV found entry to another group of people and a way to enter into the heterosexual community. While people were tuning out with drugs, they were also setting the stage for addiction to set in, and with it a dependency that could eventually drive them to behaviors facilitating HIV transmission. The following case study provides a clear example:

Case Study 3.2

Sandy is a 47-year-old mother of three. She is not HIV-positive, but has lost over six friends to AIDS. She has been a recovering addict for 18 years, since she started using heroin in 1968 while she was in college at Brandeis University.

"I thought that drugs were bad when I was growing up. My parents did not talk to me about them, really no one did. They were around, but it was not something that I thought about. I thought that pot was a bad drug when I was in high school. When I went to college, the war was starting, people were smoking grass, and I tried it. I never really got into using, never really got into drinking. I was not out of control until I started to drop acid. I would get screwed up on the weekends, but I was still in school and doing well. There were no indicators that I was in trouble. In my senior year, I snorted smack for the first time. I do not know if it was love at first, but it sure did take the edge off. The time was really stressful, people were so united against the war, that you felt that no matter what happened they would be there for you. It was okay to try drugs because people were there for you. If you had a bad trip, people would be there to get you through it. I started to shoot after I had been using smack on the weekends. The minute I started to shoot I needed the stuff, I cannot … wait" she asks me, "did you ever dive down to the drain at the bottom of a pool when you were a kid?"

I tell her yes, that I used to dive down to the drain of a pool when I was a child.

"Do you remember what it was like right before you got back to the surface, that rush to get air? That is what every day was like for me; the drug became my air, everything I did was about getting the heroin. I would do anything to get my hands on the stuff. I shared works with people all the time. I was teaching third grade at the time. I would go into the faculty bathroom and shoot up all day. No one knew, no one tried to stop me. I was shooting into my arms, legs, feet. I had infections all over my body from using dirty needles. I had hep. I am so lucky, I cannot believe I don't have HIV. The '60s and '70s were a tough time, it is hard to believe that I made it out, or for that matter anyone did. I guess that there is a price to pay. I started to go to Narcotics Anonymous in the late '70s. No one had heard of AIDS then, but now there are so many people in the room that have it, it is devastating. I am not sure what is worse—AIDS or being addicted and losing your choice. It is ironic that is what the 1960s and the entire movement was about—having the choice—and the drugs took that away faster than the government ever did. Now AIDS seems to be adding insult to injury. I am not sure how these people that are positive stay straight. To get clean and enter a new hell, it keeps me clean on the worst days that I have."

Medical Technology

The 1950s, 1960s, and 1970s brought new technology to a host of health care issues, such as surgery, emergency medicine, and transplantation of tissues. With improved technology, health care officials were therefore able to intervene in the processes of many diseases. Cancers were being treated with powerful chemotherapies that often caused anemia. Blood transfusions combated anemia, often buying enough time to get the person through a crisis and thus into a possible remission. By pooling blood (combining many people's blood donations) and isolating its components, doctors were able to give just what was needed to the patient. Those suffering from severe blood loss therefore could be given whole blood; those needing plasma alone could receive it; those needing only factor VIII could receive just factor VIII. What was not realized was that the saying "one bad apple will spoil the entire bushel" applied to blood pools. All it took was one contaminated unit to infect many patients. The need for blood products only increased with the advances that were made in modern medicine. As the demand increased, greater efforts were made to procure donors.

Computer networks had started to coordinate efforts of health care professionals. If a person needed a certain type of blood—for example, a transfusion of type AB—it might have been donated by a person across the state. With air travel available to transport blood, new chemical additives to act as preservatives, and computers to access needs, transmitting HIV no longer required that the infected person know or even be near the person who was being infected. An HIV-infected person in New York City could now infect a stranger in Buffalo.

Summary

HIV is not a new virus. What is new about it is that it has moved outside its natural reservoir. It most likely originated in Africa and through advances in travel and technology spread to other populations. The first confirmed case of AIDS was retrospectively diagnosed through PCR analysis dating back to 1952, which conclusively proves that HIV is not a new virus that originated during the 1970s and 1980s.

AIDS was first recognized in 1981 in young, previously healthy gay males in New York, San Francisco, and Los Angeles, and was called gay-related immunodeficiency (GRID), taking its name from the population in which it was first identified.

The disease was thought to be caused by many different agents ranging from semen to nitrate inhalants. In 1986, a retrovirus later known as HIV was isolated by a scientist in France at the Pasteur Institute.

The proliferation of AIDS in the United States was generally attributed to gay males and their promiscuous sexual activities. A more thorough and accurate explanation for the viral amplification encompasses both the social and the technological changes that created a more global community.

4

HIV Testing
Understanding the Science of Testing

The need for HIV testing is obvious: The only way to know for sure if a person has HIV is to test for the virus. But the psychological and societal implications of testing are extraordinary. Those who are tested need to know the difference between confidential and anonymous tests, the possibility of incorrect test results, and the proper time frame for testing after possible exposure. Deciding who should be tested and why requires that the rights of the individual be balanced against the welfare of society.

The Science of Testing for HIV

The presence of HIV is determined by culturing from blood samples and by polymerase chain reaction tests. The procedures most commonly used to ascertain a person's HIV status, however, do not test for the presence of HIV, but for the antibody. The common screening process for HIV involves the use of two laboratory tests, the ELISA and the Western blot.

The ELISA Test

The *enzyme-linked immunosorbant assay* (ELISA) test is used as the preliminary screening test because it does not pose a great risk of returning a false negative test result. The test looks for the presence of HIV antibodies in a blood sample. A blood sample is placed in a vial that has been coated with the HIV antigen. The tray is then mixed with an enzyme that links to the antibodies, which are now attached to the antigen lining the side of the wall. The trays are then rinsed again, washing out any enzyme that did not find antibodies to bind with. A substrate is added that will bind to the enzyme and cause a reaction resulting in a visible color change. If a test has this color change, it is considered positive, meaning that the person tested is thought to have HIV. Figure 4.1 illustrates the ELISA test procedure.

The reason this test is not used exclusively is that it occasionally returns a false-positive result; that is, it suggests that a person has HIV when in fact he does not. The false-positive test results occur when other viruses are present that cause the production of antibodies; these antibodies react with the ELISA in a way that is similar to HIV, and thus make it appear that HIV

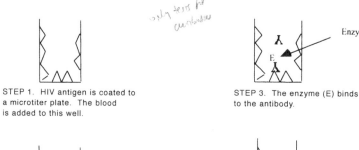

STEP 1. HIV antigen is coated to a microtiter plate. The blood is added to this well.

STEP 3. The enzyme (E) binds to the antibody.

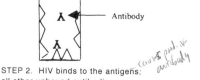
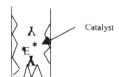

STEP 2. HIV binds to the antigens; all other unbound antibodies are washed away.

STEP 4. Catalyst is added which causes a color reaction in the presence of the bound antibody.

FIGURE 4.1. Diagrams illustrating the ELISA test that is used as the first part of an HIV antibody screening exam.

antibody is present when it is not. Such a result can occur when a person is infected with other viruses that have similar proteins embedded on the viral envelope, such as viral hepatitis. Even though false-positive results are rare, the far-reaching implications of a positive test demand that test results be accurate. To assure that the results are accurate, positive samples are tested again using another more sensitive test called the Western blot. Those results that are not positive in the ELISA test are not run through the other tests, and the person's status remains HIV-negative.

The Western Blot Test

The Western blot test is more sensitive than the ELISA test and, when coupled with the ELISA, acts as a definitive test for the presence of HIV. This test screens for specific components of HIV antibodies. The Western blot test uses a detergent to disrupt the light- and heavy-chain proteins that are located on the amino ends of the HIV (see Figure 4.3).

This process separates the proteins into their individual components. Once separated, they are sized and placed on sodium dodecyl sulfate (SDS) polyacrylamide gels. These gels are layers of a substance in which the proteins can move and find equilibrium according to their densities; the heavier proteins sink lower in the gels than the lighter proteins. By calibrating the gels, it can be determined which protein is which, as each has a molecular weight different from the molecular weights of other similar proteins. The proteins are then transferred onto sheets of nitrocellulose. The sheet is cut into strips, which in turn are incubated with samples of the blood that tested positive in the ELISA test. The strips are then washed and an enzyme label, anti–human antibody, is added. In a positive result, a visible enzyme is left behind on the strips. Figure 4.3 illustrates the Western blot test procedure.

While it is clearly very important to understand test results, it is also crucial to be able to explain what factors can influence a test result and how these factors might mislead a person from the truth about his HIV status.

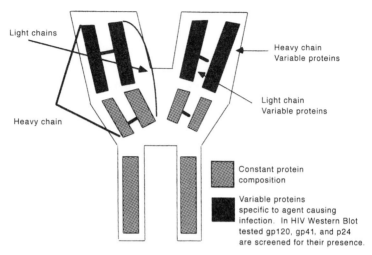

FIGURE 4.2. Antibody diagram illustrating the light and heavy chains disrupted by the Western blot test.

Interpreting the Results of an HIV Antibody Test

An ELISA test is declared HIV-negative if there is no reaction between the HIV-coated walls of the testing tray and the individual's blood sample. The Western blot test looks at the specific proteins that compose the HIV antibody: gp120, gp41, and p24. Each of these proteins is identifiable by a pattern of bands much like the familiar bar codes now in everyday use. There must be at least two of these proteins present for a test to be considered positive. If no bands are displayed, it is thought that the person is HIV-negative and that something other than HIV might have caused the ELISA test to give a false-positive result. Occasionally, some but not all of the bands are present; in these cases, the test results are considered indeterminate.

These procedures test only for the presence of an antibody, not for the presence of the virus. A negative test does not mean that the person being tested does not have HIV; it does mean that

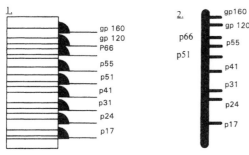

HIV is disrupted and broken down into its viral protein components by molecular weights. The process is called polyacylamide gel electrophoreisis.

The HIV proteins are now arranged on a nitrocellulose strip.

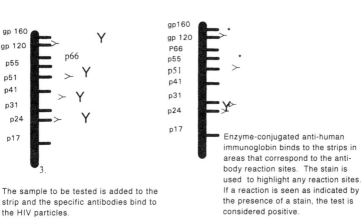

The sample to be tested is added to the strip and the specific antibodies bind to the HIV particles.

Enzyme-conjugated anti-human immunoglobin binds to the strips in areas that correspond to the antibody reaction sites. The stain is used to highlight any reaction sites. If a reaction is seen as indicated by the presence of a stain, the test is considered positive.

FIGURE 4.3. Diagram illustrating the procedure in the Western blot test, which looks at the specific protein components of HIV.

the person is not producing HIV antibodies. It usually takes a few weeks after exposure (the average being 6 weeks) for the body to produce antibodies. This period of time between infection and the production of antibodies is called the _window period_. During the window period, HIV can still be transmitted from one person to another. It is this window period that makes it impossible to guarantee the absolute safety of blood transfusions.

The Testing Process

The HIV antibody test is a process that can take up to 3 weeks from start to finish. The process begins with getting the client to recognize that he or she needs to be tested. The person seeking a test must first decide what type of test setting he or she wants. For example, a test may be obtained at a private practice, but this costs money and the test results are not as private as they can be in other settings. It is important to understand the policies that are associated with each testing process.

Anonymous Tests

Anonymous tests are usually sponsored by government agencies, such as county health departments, and are conducted in hospitals and clinics. They use a number to identify the person being tested instead of the person's name. The blood is drawn into a test tube labeled with a number, and the person being tested is asked to look at the test tube and record the number. The lack of information precludes tracing the number to a person's identity. Clinics do not give the results out over the phone; the person being tested must return to the clinic to get the results in person.

Anonymity encourages testing of people who might otherwise not be tested. The fear of having others learn one's HIV status is substantial. It is also justified, as validated by the prejudice against people with HIV regularly seen in the United States and throughout the world. When it was learned that three male children in the Ray family of Arcadia, Florida, had HIV as a result of receiving transfusions of HIV-positive factor VIII, someone set fire to their house, which burned to the ground. The family was forced to move, leaving their friends, family, and schools to avoid the tremendous negative reaction of the community.

Often, the person conducting the test is not a trained health care professional. This trend started in the mid-1980s, when there was a lack of professionals working with HIV. The shortage was addressed by training social workers and other non–medically trained people to staff testing centers. It was previously unheard of in Western society for anyone but a physician to test for, and then inform someone about, a terminal disease. This does not mean that HIV tests are invalid or that people who seek anonymous tests are putting themselves at risk. The problem is that people who are given devastating test results often have a desire to ask questions and to hear an answer from a doctor. In this setting, there is no opportunity to do so.

Another disadvantage of this type of testing is that the test results lack statistical value. There is really no way to weed out repeated tests of one person. If, in a year, one person is tested four times, and on the fourth test he comes up HIV-positive, the statistic looks as though one out of four tests is positive.

The data collected in anonymous screening tests are used by epidemiologists to track the spread of the disease in certain populations, especially drug abusers, gay men, and newborn children.

The sites that report data to the Centers for Disease Control and Prevention (CDC) and the National Institutes of Health (NIH) come from the Army, the Job Corps (a federal program that is offered as an alternative educational avenue for young people who, either as a condition of probation or parole or voluntarily, enter to learn a skill or trade), public health departments, and correctional facilities. The data are not comprehensive because most states do not record or report the numbers of HIV-positive test results, but rather the numbers of AIDS cases.

The results of the seropositive screening efforts should not be dismissed, though, because these screening tests suggest that HIV is becoming more prevalent in the general population.

According to a study conducted by the CDC, nearly 15% of all gay men who were tested in the STD (sexually transmitted disease) clinics tested positive for HIV antibodies. Drug rehabilitation centers that participate in reporting HIV status showed a 7.5% median prevalence. The rate from clinic to clinic across the country showed a variance ranging from 15% to 40%. In adolescent populations, the seroprevalence remained below 1%. This information was obtained from data collected from the Job Corps, juvenile detention centers, military records, and adolescent medical clinics. In teenage runaways, the prevalence was higher, at 2.6%, but only five youth shelters participated in this study.

Distribution of HIV according to race supports the same trends that were seen in AIDS surveillance studies. Blacks are disproportionally affected by HIV, with a median positive rate of 43.6% for black gay men compared to 23.2% for their white counterparts. Transmission caused by injection drug use was 23.2% in blacks, compared to 18.4% for whites. Black women of childbearing age were 28 times more likely than whites to have HIV. The seroprevalence statistics are similar for whites and Hispanics in the western states, but Hispanics have a higher rate of HIV in the east coast states.

The seroprevalence rates vary a great deal because of inconsistent reporting by states and communities. Different states require different information to be reported. The inconsistency is responsible for a 60-fold variation in HIV seroprevalence across different urban areas.

The screening tests are also used to monitor the safety of the blood supply. In 1985, the CDC started to collect data from donor sites. According to the CDC findings, nearly 8 million people donate 13 million units of blood per year. The prevalence of HIV in this population (blood donors) is less than in the general population because those who might be at risk for HIV are discouraged from donating blood. To date, 1 in 20,000 units of blood will be HIV positive and get past the screening tests. Blood that is found to contain HIV antibodies is destroyed.

Confidential Tests

The confidential test is not coded with a number, but is labeled with the names of the person and the physician who ordered the test. This test remains confidential, and the information from the test cannot be given to any person or agency without a written release. This precaution does not mean, however, that information will not be leaked to others. Tests that can identify an individual are handled with the same privacy safeguards as any other type of medical procedure. Tests that are given by private physicians are not free, and if a person wants his insurance company to pay for the testing costs, the insurance company might want to know the results.

The results that come from a doctor's office can be given over the phone (although doctors often tell their patients that they want them to come in for the results). The waiting time for the results is often shorter because a doctor's office usually has fewer people to test than a clinic that specializes in testing for HIV. This testing process also keeps the entire process in the hands of a physician, who is qualified to make a judgment about the current health of the person who receives a positive test result.

Helping People Recognize Reasons to Be Tested for HIV

There are people who know they should learn their HIV status even though they see their doctor and never talk about the virus. They think about an HIV testing, but do not receive one because they feel shame and fear. For some people, especially those who have engaged in risk behaviors, this type of fear is a prison. These people need help in realizing that learning their HIV status might make them feel better in the long run.

The reasons to take an HIV test are not always clear. Some people do not see the value in knowing what their status is, or they simply fear the results. Getting a person to see value in learning his HIV status is not impossible; helping a person overcome a fear of something he has good reason to fear is another situation altogether. The situation is perhaps analogous to that of people who fear a diagnosis of cancer.

Why would it be necessary to learn one's HIV status? How does this information help a person's life? The answers are simple. Learning one's HIV status is necessary if a person is sexually active. While all sexually active people whose HIV status is not known to be negative should practice safe sex, it must also be remembered that "safe sex" is not synonymous with "risk-free."

This distinction is relevant because it is a component of making an informed choice.

People are frequently unable to acknowledge that they have put themselves at risk. Rather than simply telling a person that he should take the test because he has been at risk for transmission (a fact that he probably is already aware of at some level), a better approach is to help him identify himself as having been placed at risk. The following questions are used to help the person seeking a test to identify himself as "at risk":

1. Ask the client to identify when he was first sexually active with another person. A person who began sexual activity in the 1950s, and has since not had sex outside a monogamous relationship, is not really at risk for being infected with HIV through intercourse.
2. Ask the person to list the number of people with whom he has had intercourse. The greater the number of partners, the greater the risk of having been exposed to the virus. Ask the person to state how many times, if any, he has had intercourse without using a condom.
3. Ask the person if he has used any intravenous drugs. Intravenous drug users are at an extraordinary risk of getting HIV from this behavior.
4. Ask about the people the client has been involved with, and whether any of them are IV drug users or gay or bisexual men. Help the person who is trying to decide whether to seek an HIV test to understand that even though he may not specifically know a given partner to have engaged in a particular activity, the partner may nonetheless have done so.
5. Ask the client if he has ever thought about having an HIV antibody test. Often, this is the point at which the client may being to talk about the reasons he feels such a test is necessary. Ask the client directly why he thinks being tested for HIV is necessary.

Once the information is gathered, repeat back to the client what he has reported. Do not use the information to scare the client into taking the test. Use it to help him identify some of the risks of exposure that he may have taken in the past. It is often helpful to point out to the client that having the test does not change the reality that he either has or has not been exposed to HIV. He will not be altered by the test. Some people do not see the fact that they have been at risk as a compelling enough reason to be tested; for these people, it often takes more time and gentle persuasion. "Guilting" a client into taking a test is not acceptable, and it rarely works. The human service worker or physician who wants to persuade a person to be tested must remember that the choice is the client's.

Helping the client to see why he should have the test might be a long process. There should be some explanation about the benefits of having an HIV test—for example, the ability to be proactive in avoiding infection and to make efforts to protect others. It is especially important to stress to the client that the test will lead him to one of two possible places. Either way, behavioral changes will be called for. The person whose test result is HIV-positive clearly has many issues to face. Questions and fears about the ways that HIV affects family life, friendships, and the workplace are natural and justified. What must always be explained is that foremost on the person's agenda should be getting good health care. Similarly, a negative test result raises issues the health care worker must address. News of HIV-negative status often causes a client to feel elated, relieved, and safe. The professional needs to remind the client that just a short while before, the client believed that he might have been infected. There should be some exploration of the behavior that made the client think he was at risk and some discussion about risk reduction.

It is recommended that the professional discuss with the client beforehand how the client might react if the result were positive. It is not unusual for the client to say that he will kill himself if the result is positive. Such a statement must be taken seriously. A person who is threatening to hurt himself, and has a plan to do so, is more inclined to do so. A plan has components, and it is all right to ask the client about those components. Has he tried to kill himself before? Does he have an idea of how he would do this? Does he have the ability to accomplish the act? The dynamics of the situation should also be explored: There is an inherent contradiction involved in being suicidal because death is imminent. When a person says that he will kill himself if he learns that he has a terminal disease, he is probably expressing a desire for control over his life. That is, he will not allow this disease to kill him; he will instead kill himself. The professional should help the client to make plans that will allow him to have a sense of control over how he lives with the disease. There also might be fear of suffering involved in the death process that leads one to suicidal ideation. Further exploration of these fears can often assist the HIV-positive person in sorting out the difference between anxiety over future suffering versus wanting to commit suicide.

Few people actually commit suicide upon hearing that they have the HIV infection, but there are those who do not have the strength to hear such news. In the cases in which it is apparent that a person might very well harm himself, it is better for him to be tested after he has become more stable and has no real suicidal ideation. It is best if a person returns at another time with someone who can help him handle the news.

Talking about Positive Test Results

The first conversation an HIV-positive person has about his status can set the stage for the way he will handle his sickness. The professional who discloses the test results should keep in mind the emotional and social impact of HIV-positive status. It affects self-perception and the level of confidence with which a person deals with his social environment, which will now include the health care system.

A person who has HIV will face many challenges, and without the help and support of friends and family, these challenges can be insurmountable. Culture and religion are other aspects of a client's life that should be discussed during the testing process; the more the professional knows about the client, the more helpful he can be in suggesting where the client might look for support. The health care worker should have a program to follow when disclosing positive results. The components of this program should include:

- Counseling to help the person establish links to support networks that are germane to medical care, mental health, and social functioning.
- Continued assessments for evidence of intent to do violence to either self or others.
- Examinations that evaluate and determine the stage of the infection.
- Exploration of the person's emotional support system.

The following case history reveals the experiences and feelings of a young man who went through the testing process and who talks freely about the possibility of suicide when facing a positive HIV test result:

Case Study 4.1

"When I was first tested, I went to my doctor. I had used needles for about three years before I stopped poppin'. I was never really afraid of HIV because I only used drugs on the weekends, and I only used them with a few people. But one of them got sick and called and told me it was HIV. I called my doctor about it, and he told me to come in to his office. It was funny because I was not really seeing the doctor except for a physical every other year. He was always nice, but we really did not know one another. On this occasion, he sat down with me and said that he wanted to talk to me before he took my blood to have it tested. He asked me what I would do if I were infected with HIV. I told him that I was not sure what I would do. He asked me if I would hurt myself. I told him that I would not at this point, but if I was really sick that I might think it over. He asked me about God and if I had faith. I told him that the jury was out on that one. He asked me if I had family and friends who I could talk to about this if I was infected. I told him that I thought I could. It was odd because we never really talked before this test was done."

JIMMY, 33, *bartender and artist*

It is difficult to probe so deeply into a stranger's life. An intimate bond can be created. The client feels that the health care

worker knows about significant aspects of his life, and the impact
of disclosing HIV test results can exact a high emotional price on
the worker. Workers must assure that they have adequate support
in their lives because telling people that they have a deadly disease and witnessing the resulting pain can be damaging over time.

Case Study 4.2

"I started out as a social worker. I never thought that I would end
up in an HIV clinic performing HIV antibody screening exams. I
took a course that was given by the Department of Health. The
incidence of HIV was not high in this area when I started testing
people. I had given 42 screening exams before I had to give back my
first positive result. It is a day I will never forget. This young man
came into my office. He was the sweetest, prettiest man I think that I
have ever seen. Actually, he was a young man, he was 19. He came
in to get tested because he was gay. I asked him why he thought that
he might have been exposed to HIV. He told me that he had been
sexually active for about two years with other men. I asked him
what he would do if he were to be HIV-positive, and he just looked
at me and said that he had no idea what he would do if it were
positive. We talked for a while about safe sex, and then I took a
sample of blood. He looked so frightened, he reminded me of my
son, and I will tell you I just wanted to hug this kid and not let him
go.

"About 15 minutes before he came back for his second visit to
get his results, I looked at the results to his test and saw that he was
positive. I thought I was going to split in pieces. I had no idea how I
was going to tell this sweet young thing that he had HIV. I have
never in my life experienced having information like this before. It
is a very large responsibility. It never really hit me until I saw this
test result.

"When he came into my office, he sat down and we said our
hellos. I asked him about what he might do if he were to get a
positive result. He said that he did not know, but he said that he
would not kill himself. I think he knew that this was what my fear
was, or that this is what the counselor wanted to hear. I also did not
think that this man would hurt himself. Call it a gut feeling.

"I asked him to read me his number for confirmation, and he
did. Then I told him that the test came back positive. I will never
forget the look on his face. His eyes started to well with water and
he asked me, 'This means that I have AIDS?' I explained to him that
he has the virus that causes the disease. He just sat there and looked

right at me. I asked him if he was okay. He said that he needed to sit
for a while. He sat for about 15 minutes. I never witnessed such
profound pain before. After a while he got up and pulled on his coat
and walked out the door. I remember the date, what the weather
was like, what I was wearing! After he left I went to the women's
room and got sick. I never cried like I did that night. This is not a job
for the weak, I will tell you."

SARAH, 40, *social worker*

Discussing Confidentiality

The professional involved in the testing process should discuss with the client the limits of confidentiality. The discussion
should include those times when results might be disclosed
against a person's will, as well as those instances when the person
might want to share his HIV status with others. The client should
know, for example, that states can require testing facilities to
report test results (although this is usually for statistical purposes).
Confidentiality can also be broken in cases in which it is established that other people are at risk as a result of someone's behavior and lack of disclosure.

One of the most compelling reasons to disclose one's HIV
status is to prevent the further spread of the virus. People should
be encouraged to share this information with sexual partners and
those who share drug paraphernalia. But disclosure does not
come without fear or risk. Although it is illegal to discriminate
against those who have HIV, cruelty and prejudice are nonetheless
prevalent, and sometimes the choice about whether to disclose is
taken away from the infected person.

Case Study 4.3

"I was diagnosed with HIV in my doctor's office. I had been getting
sick with pneumonia, and they were not sure what was going on. I
was married at the time, and I am a physician, so no one thought
that I might be suffering from HIV or AIDS. I had been seeing men
in anonymous places and tricking around. I really did not want to
be gay. I loved having my children and the life I had. It was just that
I really had a sexual need to be with men.

"My marriage ended, and I was becoming emotionally in-volved with a man. Then I started to get sick. Finally, they took a blood test for HIV antibody, and it came back positive, and they diagnosed me with AIDS. It had only been two years since my first gay interaction, so I never thought that I could have AIDS, and I'm a doctor. Well, in any event I was released from the hospital and went home. I told my partner and we cried for awhile. I then called my ex-wife and told her that I needed to talk to her about something. We had not been getting along that well after she found out that I was gay. I can understand, but she came, we share a bond because of our children. I told her what happened and she went ballistic. After what was the most powerfully emotional night of my life, I thought that the hard part was over.

"A few weeks later on the front page of the newspaper was the leading story: 'Pediatrician Has AIDS.' It covered my personal life, where my practice was, and the fact that I had been practicing with HIV. I cannot begin to tell you the rage that I felt. They had no right to do that to me. This is not 1981, where people do not understand what HIV is and how it is transmitted; it's 1992, for God's sake."

Том, 38, *pediatrician*

A person who learns that he or she is HIV-positive will expe-rience a severe identity change. Whereas before the test he might have thought of himself as healthy, he is now faced with being ill. It is unusual for people in their twenties and thirties to be diag-nosed with a terminal disease; younger people are particularly unprepared for it. Gathering information about doctors, hospital services, labs, and research projects must become a focal point of life.

Many people who are HIV-positive are involved with others who may also have the virus and who do not yet know it. Dis-closure can therefore be twice as difficult in that there is now knowledge that both people might be infected.

Case Study 4.4

"I found out that I was HIV-positive three years ago. My lover came home one day and was sitting in the living room. It's odd, but the moment I walked into the house I knew something was very wrong. I asked him what was wrong and he just looked at me. He never said a word, he just started to cry, and I thought that maybe a friend had died or something. He just kept saying over and over again, 'I've got it, I've got it.' I never felt so sad or scared in my entire life. The entire night we sat in that room and cried. Bruce was crazy upset. After hours of crying, he told me that he felt bad because he might have given it to me. I was tested and my results were positive. Bruce never got past the fact that he gave me the virus. I was never mad at him for infecting me after I chose to be with him. I am just mad because he left first and showed me all I have to look forward to as I get sick. We were in this together, and then he left me. It is so unfair."

TED, 34, *schoolteacher*

Summary

There are few medical tests that generate more anxiety than the HIV antibody test. The fear of the results keeps many from getting tested. The risks of not knowing one's status, however, bring people to the point where they have to deal with that fear and be tested. When a person comes into a clinic for the first time to see a counselor, it is imperative that the person who is conducting these tests have knowledge of the subject and remember that he is the introduction to a system that can be very frightening.

Tests are usually administered in one of two ways: in either a confidential or an anonymous setting. The confidential results are recorded by the person's name, whereas the anonymous test uses a number to identify the person. In most cases, the anonymous tests are free of charge, usually paid for by public health agencies.

Helping a person to recognize reasons to be tested for HIV is important and is often the approach that will help a person to freely take the test. At this point there is also the ability to give information that can be used as a method of risk reduction—that is, helping the person to act in such a way that his risk of future infection or the possibility of transmitting the virus is reduced.

Testing and getting the results of a test can take anywhere from 3 days to 3 weeks depending on the setting, with confidential tests usually being faster.

Those having an HIV test should think about the support that they might need during this process.

A person should be in a sound mental and emotional state when he receives the test results. If a person cannot ensure that he will not hurt himself, a future appointment may be a wiser choice—for both the client and the worker.

5

The Natural Course
of an HIV Infection

AIDS is by definition considered a separate disease from HIV infection, though in reality it is more of a marking post on the continuum of an HIV infection. Some people travel along this continuum at a faster rate than others. There are some who have had HIV for 2 years and develop AIDS, and there are some who have had HIV for over 10 years and do not meet the criteria for an AIDS diagnosis. Most people, however, usually start to show signs of having an opportunistic infection that characterizes an AIDS diagnosis within 7 years after their initial infection. The period of time that elapses from when a person is first infected to the point where he becomes sick was once called the "dormant" period. Researchers who had studied the disease for over a decade have shown that this is not the case—HIV is not dormant, but is kept in check by the immune system. Eventually, the immune system loses the battle to the virus and the person becomes ill, often resulting with one or more of the many opportunistic infections that signify AIDS. This period of time from infection to full-

blown AIDS is marked by subtle changes as the virus continues to
make progress against the body's defenses.

Early HIV Infection

Often described as an influenzalike illness, the early-stage
infection occurs 2–12 weeks after the first exposure to HIV. During
this time, the virus is reproducing at a high rate; in fact, there is
more virus in the blood during this time than at any other time
before the late stages of the disease set in.

After infection, it is not uncommon for there to be symptoms
that mirror those of mononucleosis. Primary HIV infection is a
complex illness that can have many symptoms. Many report a
moderate to severe fever, and other symptoms include rashes,
diarrhea, nausea, vomiting, swollen lymph nodes, sore throat,
muscle and joint aches, and severe headaches. These symptoms
usually disappear without specific treatment, because the body's
immune system will rally and be able to fight this initial infection.
These symptoms are important signs of HIV infection for those at
high risk because conventional HIV blood tests, which look for
antibodies, cannot detect infection during the initial weeks. People
do not form HIV antibodies until 2–6 months after infection,
weeks after the early, primary infection period. It is during this
time that the amount of HIV is highest in the bloodstream, making
transmission more likely if the infected person engages in risk
behaviors.

After a few weeks, most people start to feel better and usually
enter into what was previously called the "dormancy" period. It
is, sadly, a case of the battle having been won, but the war having
just started.

Midstage HIV Infection

After a person "recovers" from the early-stage HIV infection,
the only way to know the relative health of the immune system is

to look at its individual components. Looking at the levels of T lymphocytes is the primary ⁛⁙ ⁙ to evaluate this system.

Lymphocyte Counts as a Measure of Health

Those with a T-cell count greater than 600 cells/mm³ of blood should have their blood monitored every 6 months. If a count of 1300/mm³ drops to 700/mm³ over the course of 6 months, testing should be more frequent. The reason is not that a count of 700/mm³ is dangerous, but rather that the rate of decrease was so swift. However, once the count falls to a value between 200 and 600 cells/mm³, testing should be increased to every 3 months, as these levels indicate that the immune system is under duress. When the count falls below 200 cells/mm³, the person has AIDS. These T-cell levels are not necessarily indicators of how the person feels, but rather are indicators of what the immune system can fight. As the cells decrease, the body is more susceptible to infections, and as a result of these various infections the person feels sick.

T-Cell Levels and Treatment

As the level of T cells decreases, the chance becomes greater that a person will experience opportunistic infections that are in some cases preventable, such as PCP. In other cases, doctors can watch these levels and begin to prescribe antiviral therapies that lower the rates of viral production.

When T cells fall below 500 cells/mm³, there should be some discussion about the possible use of antiviral therapies that will help temporarily increase the amount of healthy T cells in the body. The most common antiviral drug used to treat HIV is zidovudine (ZDV), formerly known as azidothymidine (AZT).

Not all patients can tolerate ZDV. It is a strong medication that is too toxic for some individuals to tolerate. Moreover, those who can tolerate the drug often reach a point at which ZDV no longer helps to keep HIV in check because the virus develops a

resistance to the drug. For these two reasons, intolerance and
resistance, many people use other antiviral therapies such as didanosine (ddI) or zulcitabine (ddC).

As the T cells approach a level near, or below, 200 cells/mm^3,
intervention is warranted to prevent certain diseases that are often
extremely difficult to treat after diagnosis. The most commonly
used prophylactic therapy prevents PCP in those with T-cell
counts below 200 cells/mm^3. Trimethoprim–sulfamethoxazole
(TMP-SMX) is the most common drug combination used to prevent the onset of PCP. Other drugs used as prophylaxis against
PCP are pentamidine, diapason, and pyrimethamine.

While there are some diseases for which physicians can offer
medications to delay or prevent onset, most of the opportunistic
infections associated with AIDS and HIV infections are not preventable, eventually bringing havoc and despair to those who
have the disease. The stages that people go through emotionally
are connected with the state of their health as well as the amount
of time that has passed since their diagnosis as HIV-positive.

HIV to AIDS: The Emotional Journey

Understanding the emotional phases that a person passes
through as he becomes more aware of the disease is a key part of
working and caring for someone with HIV. Such understanding
not only removes some of the fear associated with watching a
person suffer, but also provides protection. It is not easy to watch a
person become progressively sicker, nor is it easy to care for him.
Caretakers are often the targets for the patient's rage and anger,
for no other reason than that they are there. Familiarizing oneself
with these emotions can, at the very least, help a person to understand that these feelings and their display are "normal" and not
personal. While it makes being the target no less hurtful, at times
when the stress is insurmountable, it provides comfort to know
that others have traveled the same path and that they have built
some bridges for others to walk across.

The Emotional Stages Associated with HIV

There are many who have studied loss and its effect on the heart and the mind. The feelings aroused are denial, anger, fear, acceptance, and resignation, occurring in no particular order. They are often situational; for instance, a person who is feeling very good is most likely going to feel a greater degree of acceptance than the person who is not. A person who is not feeling well is in a battle with the disease, and cannot escape its presence. The helping person faces the challenge of developing a map that will allow these men, women, and children to live the rest of their lives in the presence of such powerful emotions. For all parties involved, the challenge is daunting, and often unknown. The emotional and physical obstacles that people with HIV face are hard to recognize; more often than not, they are private, hidden, and unidentified.

There is the temptation to look for stages and develop solutions. All such solutions are predicated on the belief that people are pretty much the same and that their reactions to dying and being sick are likewise the same. It is the mantra of some, often those following the 12-step approach developed by Alcoholics Anonymous, to proclaim that we are not unique, and this "terminal uniqueness" is an emotional crutch that can isolate a person and keep him from understanding that he is not the only one affected by what he is going through. This ideology is meant to help a person keep things in perspective. Unfortunately, this idea that people are the same and pass through the same emotional stages is not always a sound approach to help the person who is suffering. The relationships that develop between people are unique to those people. They are born of opportunity, disclosure, and experience. The jobs they hold, the world they have seen, the lives they have lived make people unique. Some people go gently into that very bad night, while others rage until all the life slips from them. Some people make tremendous efforts to make life worth something; others sit back and take life in. It is these differences in experience and perspective that the caretaker has to account for and realize that the person's life, and his viewpoint, are all that he has. To "help" a person through an HIV infection is not only about caretaking and helping to forge a path through the myriad of societal regulations and systems, but often also requires allowing him to forge his own path and making sure that he keeps a sense of self. The helping person is the safeguard who protects integrity and personhood in the medical world, where the focus is often solely on physical health.

Understanding these feelings is not the end-all and be-all for the human service worker. In fact, understanding that the feelings exist and need to be acknowledged is what is really important.

Anxiety

After a person has an HIV antibody test and learns that he or she is HIV-positive, commonly asked questions are "When will I get sick?" and "How can I keep from developing AIDS?" There is no easy answer, and a person can take steps that promote better health: quit smoking, drink less alcohol, exercise, and eat right. Even taking these steps does not mean a person will stay in good health for a longer period of time, though it makes sense that a person will fare better if he takes care of himself. How, then, is a person who is HIV-positive to plan the rest of his life when he does not know when the disease will begin? The person who has HIV now faces the challenge of living in a world where he faces other people's fears, ridicule, and hatred. Coupled with this is the realization that one day in the relatively near future, he will most likely become sick with a horrific disease.

Case Study 5.1

Marybeth is 34 years old. She was by her own account a person who should never have been infected with HIV. She grew up in a family of four children and a mother and father. She is the second-born child. She has an older sister and two younger brothers. Raised as a Catholic, she went to Catholic schools and to a Catholic college. She graduated with a degree in education and met her spouse in 1982 while she was student teaching. They dated for two years and were married in 1987. Marybeth has said that her marriage was a good one and she had loved her husband deeply. He died of AIDS in

1990, yet she was not aware that he was HIV-positive until he became sick.

"In January, Mark started to have sleeping problems, and he would wake up and could not get back to sleep for hours. He would sit in the chair that was in the corner of the room and stare at the bed. It is so funny when you love someone, and he is looking at you when you are sleeping and then you wake up; it is just odd how you can sense that a person is watching you, and you respond, there is that connection. Once I woke up and I asked him, 'What's the matter?' and he said, 'Nothing, I'm just looking at you.' He was so beautiful, just sitting across the room looking at me.

"The next thing was the sweats. He would soak the bed. We would have to get up and change the sheets. It was really like nothing that I had ever seen before. By this point, we both knew that something was up with his health, and that this was not good what was happening, but neither one of us ever thought that it was AIDS. It was about a week later that Mark started to have difficulty breathing. We went into the hospital emergency room, and they told us that he had pneumonia.

"The next afternoon the doctor told me that he had AIDS. It was beyond a surreal moment for me. The horror that I felt I thought was one that was like nothing I had ever felt before, but to be honest it got a lot worse. They got Mark through the crisis, but he was never the same after the pneumonia. He was never able to really be active again. We didn't talk about things for a while. I mean we didn't talk about how he was infected or if I was the one who infected him.

"Three weeks to the day that Mark was released from the hospital, I started to get sick. I woke up in the morning with the worst feelings of nausea that I have ever experienced. I remember feeling so sad that this was happening to me so fast, that I was just going to fade away. That's, by the way, what Mark was doing. He was not dying, he was fading away. I called the doctor and told him that I was now sick. He suggested that I come in and get some tests to see how I was doing. It turned out that I was healthy as far as the blood work. I was pregnant, HIV-positive, and my husband was fading away. I loved Mark so much, but I was mad that he was sick, and I was mad because I thought that he had done something to betray our relationship. He was supposed to be getting sick, and the fact that he was sick only made me think that he did something to make himself sick. I was not sure what I wanted to do about the baby that was inside of me. I was simply not sure about anything any more. People ask me now, was I mad? There were times that I was angry in a way that I could not imagine. There were times that I was sad, and there were times that I was so scared. The odd thing was that I would flash through these emotions in minutes.

"It was April 2 when I decided that I had to talk to Mark about the baby, and talk to him about what was happening to us. I mean, we were together, but we never talked about AIDS. I would make sure to give him his meds, and I would lay down next to him and listen to his heart beat. I would think a lot about how much I loved this man. There was nothing that would ever make him leaving me easy. I walked into the sun porch where Mark was resting on the couch and I said, 'I'm pregnant.'

"The look on his face was like I wounded him, he just started to cry. Tears just ran down his face and he cried and cried. I started to cry. We cried for about an hour, just cried together. Finally, sitting in the door jamb holding hands, we decided that this baby could not come into this world. There was no reason to bring a child into this world, where the only thing that we could provide this baby was with pain and sadness. This should have been one of the happiest days of our marriage, and instead it was nightmare. As a Catholic, I was raised to think that abortion was wrong, a murder, but the fact was that I could not even take care of myself and Mark, let alone a baby. I had an abortion three days later. Two days later, Mark and I got a phone call from the mother of a woman that Mark used to date in college. She told us her daughter had died of a drug overdose. She was apparently a junkie since she and Mark were in college. Mark knew that she was wild, but he never knew that she was shooting dope and coke. It was like, thanks a fucking lot, lady."

This case illustrates the many repercussions that AIDS brings to a person's life. The process that each person goes through is never the same, because personal situations are different. During the interviews that were conducted to write this book, there were many different situations, but there were also some very common emotional responses that people reported, and while many of the reactions were similar, the methods used toward a resolution were never the same.

Self-Blame

Of the more than 220 people who were interviewed, 82% blamed themselves for becoming HIV-positive. All the respondents who stated that they felt responsible had contracted the virus either from unprotected sex or from using drugs. This could be interpreted as an internalization of society's early idea of the "innocent victims" paradigm. Those adults who became infected through blood transfusions, or children born to infected mothers, were thought to be innocent. Those who contracted the disease through sexual acts or the use of injection drugs were thought to be responsible for their infection. The following case study illustrates this reaction to learning that one is HIV-positive:

Case Study 5.2

"I was pretty promiscuous when I was younger. I knew that AIDS was an issue, and I knew that there were certain things that I should not have done being gay and living in New York [City]. I was tested a lot, every time after I would have what I could refer to as an encounter. Every time that I was told that I was negative I would swear that I was never going to trick again, and sure enough, after this I would go out and start to have sex with men I didn't know. I knew that it was not a healthy behavior, and I really didn't like not being in love with the men I was sleeping with. Who am I kidding— it would have been nice to know their names! I was getting depressed about what I was doing, but it was like I couldn't stop. I got this therapist who thought that I had a sexual addiction. I started to get it together and I stopped tricking around, but by then, after going through the therapy, I know that I was sleeping around because I really didn't like myself, and by then I had stopped sleeping around because I did like myself, and that's when I started to really be afraid of getting tested for HIV.

"My therapist thought that I needed to be tested if I really did care about myself and wanted to be responsible sexually. I mean it made sense that I should know my HIV status if I really wanted to get involved with another man. Well, I made an appointment to get tested and I went.

"I remember praying to my 'higher power' and really wanting to be HIV-negative. I was sure that this time I could really care for myself and value my HIV-negative status. Well, it didn't happen. I was diagnosed HIV-positive that day. Man, it sucked, and deep inside me I knew that I was to blame for this, that is, I had just done the right thing because it was right. I mean, I guess I can have a therapist tell me till I am blue in the face that I am a sex addict and I needed to get into a healthy place emotionally before I could stop, but the bottom line is I think that I fucked this up like I have fucked up a lot of things. I mean, I wish I could of been like the regular people, the ones that took the high road. I mean guys like you who go to school and learn. All I did was party and screw around and now it is all catching up with me."

DENNIS, 33, *actor and waiter*

The roots of self-blame come from the message that AIDS is a disease that can be prevented. Society's message to those who contract AIDS is: "You should have known better."

There are certain aspects of life that make it worth living; however, a world that is void of tenderness, affection, sexuality, and risk is a life that most would not find fulfilling. To combat this sense of emptiness, people take risks. This is not necessarily a bad thing, but in the age of AIDS there is an extraordinary price. It might even be that some of the behavior that puts one at risk for AIDS is understandable, even desirable, but such a conclusion does little to really help the person who suffers. It is also an effective illustration of society's prejudice toward HIV and those who are infected with the virus. There are few diseases that apply so much blame to the person who suffers. For example, there is plenty of research suggesting that smoking is unhealthy, but such knowledge does not limit the care and empathy given to those who have lung cancer and heart disease caused by smoking cigarettes. As a society, we have felt that those affected with disease are deserving of care and compassion simply because they are sick; rarely is the etiology of the disease used as the criterion by which the suffering person is deemed to deserve or not to deserve compassion and care.

As a society, we challenge this tenet when the disease is AIDS. This challenge manifests itself in a blame assessment that trickles down from policy and rhetoric to the individual, who in turn blames himself for getting the disease. The results of self-blame can be self-destructive behavior, depression, self-hatred, and loss of self-esteem. Helping a person to see that most people engage in behavior that might not have a good outcome can be helpful. The person who feels he did this to himself needs time to recover from the diagnosis, but this does not mean he will stop blaming himself.

Providing education will help some people, but some will continue to blame themselves. Constant reassurance from counselors can help relieve some of these feelings.

Most people have fears but are not gripped by their fears. Oftentimes, when a person is gripped by fear, the fear is an irrational one, a phobia. However, there are also those who have fear that is entirely rational. Many of the people interviewed reported not just that they felt fear, but that their fear was more of a backdrop against which they saw their entire world.

Case Study 5.3

Scott is a 30-year-old male who has had AIDS for 3 months. He had known that he was HIV-positive for 2 years before he got sick.

"I have lived with fear now for about 3 years. I was afraid of the virus at first, afraid that I would get it. That is when the fear started. I was afraid of AIDS and HIV way before I knew that I was positive. When I found out that I was positive, I bugged and started to be afraid of everything. Man, I was afraid that I was gonna get germs from people. I was afraid that people would not like me any more. It is sick, man. I am afraid of so many things I cannot even tell anyone about it. I get afraid that I will get sick and have a lot of pain. I am afraid that there is nothing else out there for us once we die. I just have fear. It is something that goes with HIV. It used to be real bad. I used to think that I would never get used to the feelings, but today they are a part of my life the same way that other feelings are. I guess I am learning to roll with a lot more than I was able to in the past."

Fear is a draining emotion that pulls much out of the people who experience it. It is an emotion that is not discussed. Emotions such as anger, love, and anxiety are often talked about and openly expressed; fear, however, is something that is rarely looked at and explored. Fear is a magical emotion that levels people in a way that few emotions do. Most people, independent of wealth, education, and spiritual values, are afraid of pain and death. The fear of death, and its mystery, causes people to retreat to the more mythical corners of the mind. Death is steeped in ceremony and tradition, and it is a subject that many do not like to talk about.

Ironically, death is where we are all heading. Churches, temples, and mosques are all geared to deliver the person to someplace else after the physical life is gone. But rarely is there discussion about the journey itself. To find comfort in religion or a belief in life after death requires that a person have faith. Faith is a funny thing—it is called upon rarely, and it is called upon only for limited amounts of time. Faith without challenge is something a bit less than faith, and so it is faith that, through its power, gets people through the real challenges that shake both their concepts of self in the world and the perspectives that allow them to appreciate the former.

It is this concept of faith, as a time-limited solution to tremendous stress, that AIDS challenges. Without faith that things can get better, one is left facing the bleak reality that things are going to get worse, and it might be a long, painful process. What is felt is fear, fear of leaving that which is wonderful in its familiarity, and comforting in its consistency, fear of leaving one's life, and in the process being keenly aware that before death comes, the fearful person will transform into something that others will no longer recognize.

Hyper Life

Case Study 5.4

Mary, a 37-year-old black woman, reported that after she got through the shock of being HIV-positive, she felt that she had to "live her life to the fullest." She tried to cram as much as she could into every hour of her day, and when all was said and done, she went on seven trips, hang-glided, windsurfed, listened to the vibes in Sadona, and visited more museums than she could remember.

"I just wanted to make sure that I was doing all that I could to insure that I got my money's worth of this life. I just thought that I should do more, that's all. I just thought that there should be more life under my belt before I got done with life at all."

Mary's story is not unusual. Many people whom I interviewed reported that they had to do something more with their lives before they died. They expressed a need to get things in, because they were being denied the future to do such things. Often, the activities that they would normally have been involved in before were venturesome ones such as skydiving and travel.

There are other aspects of the "hyper life" syndrome: emotional risk taking, extravagant purchases, and the desire to contact people and resolve issues that have yet to be resolved. While these are all important parts of keeping control of life, and living a good life, it is the extreme degree that is employed. The hyper life syndrome is not a "cost-free" trip. The sheer volume of emotional energy that is cycled through a person in pursuing such a lifestyle generates a tremendous swirl of feelings, emotions, and desires that can bring a person to his knees once the hyperactive capability is exhausted. As with most extremes, the body and mind can endure them only for a certain time, after which the individual is left drained.

Case Study 5.5

"My father and I did not get along when I was growing up. He's an alcoholic, and he used to drink all the time when we were growing up. It was really bad. When I was 16, he found me in bed with another guy and told me to get out of his house. I stayed with a friend for awhile, then I tried to move home. Things were good for about two days, and then he started to drink again. It was a nightmare. He started in again, calling me a faggot son, and a homo.

"I left that night and moved into a shelter. I started tricking to get money so I could eat. I hated what I was doing, it was the worst feeling that you could imagine, so I started to get fucked up because I was so unhappy about what was goin' on. Man, I would have these old guys comin' up to me and wantin' me to give them a blow job for fifteen bucks. Man, I needed to get high before that. I was out trickin' one night and this guy comes up to me, and I was really high out of mind, and I ask the guy if he's looking for some action, and WHAM the cuffs are on. I was busted for soliciting and possession.

"I was only 16, so they called my dad. He comes and takes me home, and starts to beat me up. I was black and blue. So this is it, man, I leave in the middle of the night and go to New York. Started in with the same old shit, man, sellin' my ass, and getting fucked up. By this time I am shooting up, drinkin' to come down. Then WHAM, one night I get busted again. I get told it is either a stay in Rikers or a trip to this therapeutic community, so I say fine, I'll go there

"So I get clean, go back to school, and get my GED. I got a job and started doing well. I just turned 23 when I saw this purple little spot on the bottom of my foot. Well, I guess I knew what it was, but I had never been tested for HIV. I was too afraid because of all the shit I had done. I went to the doctors and I got AIDS, just like I thought. Well, I was in AA and everything and was thinking about calling my father anyway. I heard that he was not drinking any more, and I thought that this might be a good thing to do. So I call him up and we start talking and I am thinkin' that maybe he is not as bad as I think he is, and then I ask him if he wants to get together and he says, 'Maybe.'

"We hung up the phone and I decided to write him a letter and tell him that I have AIDS. I never heard back from him. It really got me upset. This is the only family that I really have, and he wants nothing to do with me. I went through some other stuff too with a few boyfriends, it was a nightmare. Now I know that I don't have to fix my life, but I thought when I first found out that I had AIDS that I had to fix it all right away. I thought that I needed to get it all right so that I could live the rest of my life in peace. Man, I wouldn't know peace if it came up an' bit me in the ass."

GLENN, 26

Why Bother

As overwhelming as life can be, retiring from it is far more draining. The rush to find resolution, completeness, and comfort can be so daunting that it should come as no surprise that a person might get to the point where he feels that there is no point, and why bother when the end result is death. This reaction resembles depression, but there is a subtle difference. The person who is experiencing depression cannot see his way clear of the dark times to know that life presents endless opportunity. The person with the "why bother" feeling is capable of seeing that life gets better, but does not always see himself or herself as part of the picture when things do get better. This feeling is seen clearly in the following interview of a 38-year-old recovering drug addict named Wendy:

Case Study 5.6

"I know that some day there is going to be a cure for this disease, but it's just that I am not going to be here when the cure arrives. I think a lot about making changes in my life because I think that it is going to be worth it, to some degree, but then I figure why? I know that I should stop smoking, but I think that it really does not matter all that much, you know. I mean I have KS, I have like 3 T cells, I am going to die. I know that I am going to die. People think that I am depressed, and that is not the case. I just don't have all that much hope left at all. It makes you look at things differently. I am not the same person, and I don't think that there are that many things left in this world that I can change or control."

When working with a person who is in this state of mind, the natural response is to want to get him out of his "slump." This is not a slump, and to assume that it is is to take the first step down the wrong path. For some people who have AIDS, this is their perspective, the point from which they view their lives, and it does not have to be changed. It is not always pleasant to watch a person slip into a place that is devoid of hope, but for some, this is simply the place where they are. Being in such a state does not mean that a person does not have the ability to have a good time, or experience happiness, peace, and joy; it is just that these feelings occur in the absence of hope. It may not be what one normally thinks of as a healthy state of mind, but it is, after all, a realistic one.

Working with people who are experiencing these emotions can be very draining. There is an edge to working with people who experience emotions and situations through a time-limited lens. Imagine knowing that another person's life is coming to a close and the heightened sense of being and emotion that such knowledge brings. It brings to most a hint of what such an existence is like, and this usually brings anxiety and a powerful desire to "fix" the person who experiences such a perspective. Nevertheless, there is nothing wrong with such feelings and perspectives, and they do not need to be fixed, repaired, or resolved. ✓

Getting Sick

Illness for the HIV-positive person is never a minor thing. For the person who is HIV-positive, a cold that has nothing to do with being sick from HIV is difficult. Every attack on the immune system is considered to be another arrow that attacks that armor. Every sickness is a reminder that the person is not well, that this is just a hint of the onset of full-blown AIDS. AIDS is progressive, as are many of the opportunistic diseases that attack the person without an immune system.

Case Study 5.7

"When I first got sick, it was the worst, because it was when I really started to realize completely that I was not going to be able to pretend that AIDS was not an issue. I started to realize that AIDS was going to finish me off. It was a real milestone. I started to see little white patches in my mouth, and I knew that it was thrush. I was crushed. I thought, 'It's here.' "

SARA, 33, *paralegal*

The person with HIV will experience small changes in his body and the way he feels during the early course of the infection, that is, before the onset of AIDS.

Case Study 5.8

"I was starting to get sick before I had AIDS. I mean, I was having colds and fevers—all that stuff—before I was diagnosed with AIDS. I knew that I was starting to get sick about a year before I met the criteria for AIDS."

PATRICK, 40, *designer*

For some people, the response to becoming sick for the first time with an HIV-related illness is a call to arms; they react with a powerful urge to fight the virus and the disease with every part of their being. For others, it is yet another sign that they are succumbing to disease. These feelings and reactions are not separate, but exist inside the person, creating a dichotomized reaction to illness. Many of the people reported that this was the time when they felt a more pressing need for peace, often allowing things to slip away that were once important to them, but that now seemed extraneous and not worth spending energy on.

The Shrinking World

There is a response to fear that has been called "flight or fight" and that describes the action taken by most beings when they are face to face with whatever their demons might be; either they run blindly in panic, or they stand and fight the demons.

Case Study 5.9

"I was waiting for AIDS for a long time. When I was HIV-positive, I had a hard time concentrating over the past few years. I was really caught up in being HIV-positive. I filled every minute of the day. When I got sick I started to relax a little, like at least it was here, there was nothing more to fear, no more waiting ... the feeling of impending doom. I felt more comfortable not doing things. I am not sure if I am tired, and now rationalize away my freedom by saying that it's less important, but in some ways it is. I feel that I really have to tend to this part of my life. I know that it is the end and I just want to appreciate my world as long as I can. I don't need to be distracted and entertained. I'm leaving, and that is something that is really beyond. I wonder where things are going to be with me in a month, a year. I just need to be with myself."

ROBIN, 27

The person who is becoming ill with AIDS will also begin to "look" sick, and this is often another factor that causes a person's world to shrink, be it the reaction he sees from others, which is often shock, or the new face he sees in the mirror. As a person's physical image begins to change, so does his perception of self.

Case Study 5.10

Andrew is a 32-year-old attorney who has AIDS-related lymphatic cancer.

"Before this happened, this is what I looked like," he says as he passes a photograph. He appears about 180 pounds in the picture, which is the perfect weight for his 6-foot frame. Andrew has lost 40 pounds due to the complications of AIDS and the effects of chemotherapy. His hair appeared in the picture to be thick and wavy brown; now it is dry, thin, and gray. His eyes are dark and heavy, and he has lost most of his teeth. "I really never thought of myself as anything but this," he says, holding out the picture. "I guess I had to get used to being something that was not easy to look at. I don't remember when I crossed that line where people cannot recognize me. But it just got too hard to go out and see people. It was hard on them, and that makes it hard on me."

As the person with AIDS deteriorates from being a healthy person, so do the roles of friends and loved ones in this person's life. Whereas once the social constellation was composed of peers, now no one is a peer. The very things that make a group "peers" are the abilities and experiences that people share in common. The ability to be self-reliant and independent is diminished. Long-term goals are different not only in content, but also in time frame. Daily activities also define peer groups. For most people affected with AIDS, the activities that are shared are career, child-raising, and other processes that define the start of adult life. The changes of time eventually bring peer groups to a point where they support one another through age and physical deterioration, but those in their 20s, 30s, and 40s are not usually in the stage of life to need such support skills. When a peer begins to die, it brings up questions about mortality that are not always ones that a person wants to consider when he is in the fullness of life. Just as the person who has AIDS feels that he often must retreat, so too do those who are affected by the disease through a loved one.

It would be nice if there were some programs that could rectify this reaction to AIDS, or steps that could be taken to limit exodus from a person's world, but the fact remains that AIDS is a disease that scares people—and they run, take flight, and mourn.

Case Study 5.11

 "My brother was gay, though we never talked about his sexuality. It was more like something that we all knew about, but never mentioned. When he was in college, he moved to New York and never moved back upstate. When he was beginning to get sick, we all pretended that there was nothing wrong with him, but as time went on it was hard to pretend. I went down and saw him once, and I knew that he wanted to talk about it, I mean AIDS and being gay. I don't know, at the time it just seemed that we spent so much energy pretending that everything was all right that when the opportunity came to get past all that, I just couldn't rise to the occasion. I remember coming home on the train the week before Chris died, and I was thinking, 'Why do I put myself through this? Why not just talk about what is happening?' But we just could not talk about AIDS, homosexuality, and because we couldn't talk about this, there was really very little that we could talk about."

BARB, 34

As the disease progresses, the person becomes more and more debilitated. The opportunistic diseases weaken the body to such a degree that daily living skills are diminished and the person requires more and more custodial care. This often means that trained medical personnel must be available to administer treatment and care for the person. The costs of these services are often staggering and cause yet another strain. For those who can afford to have these services in the home, the setup of the house must be changed to accommodate the comings and goings of nurses and aides. The changes that occur are yet another reminder of how the person's world changes.

Case Study 5.12

"I was just diagnosed with AIDS, but I'm still feeling well. I just have a low T-cell count. I had a friend die of AIDS. They moved his hospital bed into his house, right into the living room. I don't want that to happen with me. I don't want to have everything change for AIDS, but I guess that I know it will."

TEDDY, 35

Once the person has AIDS and starts to show infections, the treatments that he has to endure can be as debilitating as the disease itself, and the combination of the disease and the treatments leaves a person often feeling washed out, tired, and forgetful. The parts of the personality that are most endearing are often the first ones to retreat deep inside the person.

Case Study 5.13

"Ryan was the most attractive man that I ever knew, both inside and out. He was my most favorite person. We lived together for six years. I remember moments when he would get me to laugh so hard that I thought I'd bust a gut. When he first got sick, we struggled to keep things together. Then he got real bad, I mean sick. The AZT was more than he could handle, but he kept trying to take it. He really did not want to die, he never wanted to give up. We had this ritual. I would get up and make coffee, and we would drink it together at the kitchen table. March 8, 1990, I got up and made the coffee. I called him, which I never had to do before, and I remember thinking a bad feeling. I walked into the bedroom, and he was sitting there in the bed crying. I asked him what was wrong. He had a fever the past few days, and was on several drugs to combat the fever. On that morning, he woke up and could not see out of his left eye. After that, nothing was the same. I never heard him laugh again. He died 6 weeks later. He died piece by piece, and when all was said and done I was left with the memory of him dying this way, and that really sucks."

FRANK, 38, *veterinarian*

As a person's world becomes more and more affected by HIV and AIDS, there are many aspects of life that are often forgotten about by helping people, doctors, and friends. A person who had AIDS or is HIV-positive still has many of the emotional needs and wants that he had before he was sick.

Sex and Illness

Many areas of the life of a person with HIV infection are looked after by health care professionals. Diet, exercise, and medicines are often the easy areas to address. The difficult areas tend to be the same areas that pose problems for people to openly discuss when they are healthy. Sexuality and sexual behaviors are important to discuss with the person who is HIV-positive. The feelings that are associated with sex are often guilt and shame. For the person who has HIV, there is also fear associated with sex.

Case Study 5.14

"After I was diagnosed with HIV, I was not really into having sex. It was like I was not sexual anymore. I was not in the mood to talk about it. I guess that I thought that it was something that was just so bad that if I did anything about it I might hurt Karen, and that was something that I didn't want to do. I knew that there were things that we could do that would not put her at risk, but I was just not into it at the time. After Karen was tested and she was negative, I felt a lot better. We had always been real afraid of getting pregnant, so we used condoms before all of this came down, but we would have oral sex and HIV can be transmitted this way, and there were times when we did not always use condoms. That is one thing that HIV has done is take out the spontaneity. We used to have sex all over the place, like we've done it in the woods and stuff, but all that ended. We have sex now, but it has to be planned more than it used to because of HIV. I mean, there are no more times that we go hiking and think that it would be fun to do it at the spur of the moment. I tell ya, all those people that think that sex is so great and that a condom spoils the mood, they do not know what a mood spoiler is! We started to have sex again after about three months. I was really nervous, and I still am. I think all the time, 'What if Karen gets it because we are doing this?' It has an effect, both good and bad. I mean, now our love making is very emotional, and it is a shared thing in a very serious way. I go to a support group, and I know that many of the people there do not engage in sexual behaviors. It is a real personal choice, and there is a lot of baggage that goes with it."

KERBY, 35, *married for six years*

Sex, for most people, is an act of significance not only because of the physical pleasures, but also because there are emotional needs that are being acted out and satisfied during the actual act. Sex expresses intimacy, caring, and love. These are feelings and endearments that a person needs when he is ill, and the person who has HIV or AIDS is no exception. Because of the long period of time between being HIV infected and the appearance of the disease (AIDS), there are sexual needs, and they should be acknowledged. It is important to realize that when a person is denied his sexuality, he might feel that he is not being viewed as a whole person. To ignore the sexuality of a person who has AIDS is particularly inappropriate. AIDS is a disease that is sexually transmitted, and there is a connection between the feelings of guilt and shame that are often associated with AIDS, similar to the feelings that are often a part of a person's sexual history. The person who has AIDS or HIV needs to understand that the powerful and good feelings that come from sex can still be experienced. There are certain steps that can be taken to ensure that sex acts are safer than if they were performed without protection, but a person still must understand that there is some risk for HIV transmission when using a condom. Ultimately, persons who are infected and their partners need to make the choices that address sexuality, sex acts, and other methods of expressing this important aspect of being human. The actual information that prescribes safer sex is discussed in Chapter 8.

Summary

There is a tremendous gray area in the treatment and care of people who are HIV-positive, but are not yet considered to have AIDS. Many of the people who are in this population experience many difficulties in many areas of their lives. These men and women are often physically healthy, but suffer from tremendous anxiety in connection with becoming sick with AIDS. Telling family members and making plans are often difficult for the person who has HIV, but they are often necessary components of having HIV.

People working with people who are HIV-positive face the extraordinary task of helping the HIV-positive person to gain perspective and turn what was once a life that was not thought to be infected with HIV into becoming a vital person who does have HIV. This is done by helping the person restructure his life, incorporating HIV as a part of his life, not the whole of it. This is done in a variety of ways, but needs to be done in a tailored and comprehensive manner that includes all aspects of the person's life: professional, social, sexual, and spiritual. Most important, it is during this time that a person has to experience life as fully as possible before he or she comes down with AIDS.

6

Medical Treatments and Those Who Administer Them

Those who have AIDS face one medical crisis after another. By virtue of the many diseases that may attack the body, the person with AIDS often has to go to specialists in order to take care of the many possible infections. Thus, health care professionals must have a good referral list to accommodate the person who needs care. For those involved in the care of AIDS patients, the profusion of specialists makes it difficult to know who does what. Who are these men and women who care for HIV-related infections? Understanding their training and limitations is a helpful aspect of working with people who have HIV infections. The same is true of medications—to understand these drugs and the way they work is to understand another piece of the AIDS puzzle.

Early in the AIDS epidemic, there was not a lot that a person diagnosed with AIDS could do. There were no treatments available for many of the opportunistic infections that attacked the body, and the virus had yet to be identified. Without a definite disease to fight, people turned to faith healers, spiritual leaders, holistic medicine practitioners, and a host of other alternative treatments. AIDS brought many of these different therapeutic approaches to the forefront of society. Today, many people use

these therapies as a primary form of treatment, while others use
parts of alternative therapies, such as relaxation and herbal teas, in
conjunction with traditional Western medical therapies. The degree of effectiveness of each form of therapy is often hotly con-
tested. When all is said and done, the individual makes a choice,
and it is the choice that needs to be preserved. How is the person
with limited knowledge to make a decision about these approaches without information? The job of explaining the differences is often left to human service workers, thus making it necessary for all people working with people to know the different
aspects of medical philosophies.

Most of those who have HIV or AIDS are young to middle-
aged people, with the average age being under 42. People in this
age group do not usually get chronically ill, nor are they socialized
to accept the possibility of chronic illness. Most simply visit a
doctor when they are sick. Medicine, in American society, is a
reaction to illness, not a method of ensuring good health. The
result of this reactive as opposed to proactive mind set is that most
people have insufficient knowledge of medicine, the variations
thereof, and available treatments to make an informed choice.

There are not only different treatments for HIV, but also
different philosophies followed in employing these treatments.
Allopathic medicine, the medicine practiced by doctors who earn
the Doctor of Medicine (M.D.) degree, has always been the standard for most Americans. For many, however, the concept of the
body and spirit being treated separately is unacceptable. Learning
about the types of medicine available simply offers a person more
options so that he may find an acceptable treatment provider.

Medical Philosophies

Most physicians are medical doctors and, like most trained
professionals, are products of their education and experience. It is
impossible to know what life experiences might be influencing a
person's perspective, but it is possible to understand the training
process that doctors go through. Medical school training is based

in science, and only recently have there been efforts to improve the curriculum, specifically to train doctors to be more empathic toward their patients. Harvard Medical School, ranked as one of the three top medical schools in the world, has changed its curriculum to allow for more patient contact in the first two years of medical school. This program, called "New Pathways," was featured on the PBS series "So You Want to Become a Doctor?"

Allopathic Medicine

The curriculum in most medical schools consists of two phases: scientific training and clinical skill development. The scientific training demands detailed knowledge of the normal structure and function of the human body and the effects of disease. This part of medical school, that is, the "classroom" part of the training, lasts for two years. Students in their first two years study for two semesters per year, with the summers off. Most of the students use these vacations to study for the boards, which are the medical competency exams that are given after the first two years of medical school. Students take gross anatomy, biochemistry, histology, embryology, and many other courses before they enter into the hospitals and begin working with patients.

The clinical training in medical school occurs during the last two years. The student spends most of his time in hospitals working with doctors and seeing in people the things that he has studied in the classroom. During this part of his education, a student will be "on rotation," spending successive 6-week periods working with doctors in areas of medicine such as pediatrics, surgery, and other specialties.

After these four years, the student graduates with the M.D. degree. At this point, the person goes on to a residency, in which he will "apprentice" in a specific area of medicine under the supervision of a specialized department.

Medical school is very competitive. Those wanting to become physicians must have strong academic records. Students admitted to medical schools have given up a great deal of their lives simply to get in and have maintained a grade point average of at least 3.5 through four years of college. These people have given up a lot to be the best in their class, often at an age when they could have been establishing a social life.

Case Study 6.1

"My dad is a doctor, and I grew up knowing all about medicine. I knew that I wanted to be a doctor, I liked the concept of it all, but I was not really ready to give up all that I had to in order to get in. I saw all of my friends going out and having fun, but I felt that I had to stay in so that I could get the grades that I needed so that I could get into medical school. Oh, I was 20 when I was feeling this way ... I was a kid. I watched them all grow up. I was too busy studying organic chemistry and physics to have the time to grow up. I was thirty years old before I had time to look back on things. I remember one reunion with all my old college friends, and they were all talking about the good times, and every good time they talked about I was not there. Frankly, medical school takes a lot of human out of you, and it also makes you give up a lot."

SCOTT, 34, *orthopedist*

There are also physicians called *osteopaths* who are trained in a different philosophy called *osteopathy*.

Osteopathic Medicine

In 1882, Andrew Taylor Sill organized the American School of Osteopathy in reaction to the primitive conditions and surgical techniques he had observed during the American Civil War. The emphasis was on treating the whole person, not just the "sick" part of the individual, and this tenet has remained an ideal of the osteopathic profession to this day. Osteopathic medicine is based on the belief that the body will manufacture its own remedies and defenses against disease if the musculoskeletal structure is in correct mechanical adjustment.

To earn the degree of Doctor of Osteopathy (D.O.) in the United States, a student must complete a three- to four-year post-graduate course of study in one of 15 recognized osteopathic colleges, and a period of hospital internship and residency is also required. Students learn to recognize structural problems, how these problems can affect the function of body organs, and how ~~chiro~~ they can be corrected through the manual manipulation of bones, muscles, ligaments, and nerves, sometimes in combination with standard medical treatments.

All states issue licenses to qualified osteopaths to practice medicine, and osteopathic institutions are accredited by the American Osteopathic Association (AOA).

While these medical philosophies are the two that are embraced by most Americans, there are other therapies that are centuries old, and still practiced all over the world. Many of them look beyond the wellness of the body to that of the spirit as well. This concept of inclusion is referred to as *holism*.

Holistic Medicine

The concept of holism was introduced by Jan Christian Smuts in 1925 as an alternative to the prevailing logical and reductive train of thought.

The holistic philosophy has slowly crept into medicine. Doctors could see that patients in more pleasant surroundings healed faster. Those working with the elderly found that having a pet could brighten a person's outlook. These observations led to the slow filtering of holism into medicine.

There are three basic aspects of the holistic approach to medicine. First, it emphasizes disease prevention by placing responsibility with the individual to use his own resources to promote health, prevent illness, and encourage healing. Holistic medicine also considers the person an individual, not as a symptom-bearing organism. Finally, holistic practitioners make use of many available diagnostic, treatment, and health methods, including both alternative and standard medical methods. Holistic health practitioners view standard medical practices as only one way to achieve good health.

The holistic health movement has gained increasing popularity and acceptance, especially in the AIDS community. The probable reason is that some of the first alleged AIDS drugs, such as the Chinese cucumber, known as Compound Q, were thought of as holistic and natural. Unfortunately, some nonmedical holistic practitioners made extravagant claims for the effectiveness of one herb or another against HIV. These so-called and often self-proclaimed "healers" have generated much criticism of the holistic philosophy, which many feel is a front for medical quackery. While the holistic approach to medicine is undergoing development and change, it is still based upon the early concept of holism first presented by Smuts.

Holistic medicine does not have one widely used diagnostic procedure or treatment because it is an attitude about health and healing. Thus, traditional physicians, nurses, specialists, and other health care professionals can consider themselves holistic practitioners. Holistic medicine addresses not only the person, but also the person's environment, involving various healing and health-promoting practices. Holistic practitioners believe that patients should be active in their own health care and thereby help to heal themselves.

Other health practices concerned with the whole person are not in themselves necessarily holistic medical practices. For example, while acupuncture involves care for the entire body, it does not include other treatments sometimes considered in holistic treatment. Acupuncture may be one of many techniques considered in holistic medical treatment. Others include biofeedback, meditation, modern fluid replacement, ancient energy balance, and surgery.

Holistic diagnosis may include standard laboratory tests or other diagnostic methods. The interrelated physical, mental, and spiritual capabilities of the whole person are major health determinants. For example, a holistic practitioner may watch the way a patient sits, stands, and walks, as well as look for the physical expression of an emotional state. Treatments are usually provided in the context of the patient's culture, family, and community.

Although holistic practitioners make use of available technical equipment and statistical analysis, the emphasis is on each patient's genetic, biological, and psychosocial strength and uniqueness. Holistic practice is designed to mobilize the individual's self-healing capacity.

Surgical or medical intervention is not disputed in holistic medical practice. Rather, the emphasis is on preventive self-care ✓ and self-education.

Holistic medicine views health as a positive state, not as the absence of disease. Such a positive approach to treating existing disease is currently being used by many researchers and physicians. This positive-attitude approach to medical care has been used in cancer therapy by having patients think differently and positively about chemotherapy and radiation therapy.

The use of touching is another major element of holistic medicine. Many body therapies, including massage, chiropractic manipulation, and rolfing (a form of massage), are dependent on physical contact. These touch-oriented therapies are based on a holistic approach to human functioning. Touch is used for greater relaxation, to improve body alignment and functioning, or to enhance awareness.

Another holistic health therapy called *psychotherapeutic body work* was first developed by Wilhelm Reich. Once an illness has been identified, it is viewed as both a misfortune and an opportunity for discovery. Holistic medicine emphasizes the idea that psychosocial stress, such as unemployment, divorce, or the death of a close relative or friend, may contribute to ill health.

In recent years, a variety of traditionally trained medical professionals have examined the ideals and documented benefits of holistic medicine. Some who see their role as counselors and healers, as well as technologically trained practitioners, embrace the humanistic approach offered by the holistic philosophy.

Folk Medicine

Folk medicine throughout the world appears to have many similar features. The body, it is thought, must have a balance of hot and cold, moist and dry, and internal and external pressure. If these balances are disturbed, the result is disease. This is expressed today every time a mother cautions her child not to go out in the cold air after a hot bath for fear of illness. The child must not walk barefoot outside before warm weather for the same reason.

The healing practices of the American Indians and the Chinese, as well as those of various cultures, properly belong to the field of ethnic medicine or anthropology. But the basic similarities of these systems to the early medicine of the Western world, and their affinities with today's Western medicine, have also made them a part of the study of folk medicine. Well into the 20th century, American Indians, for example, used incantations, or songs, to help drive out the demons of disease. Herbal medicines were also used, sometimes with magical practices, sometimes alone. Many of the herbs used by the American Indians—such as datura, coca, cinchona, curare, cascara sagrada, and the like—are now used as drugs in modern scientific medicine.

Chinese medicine has also continued many traditional practices. Most of the knowledge of early Chinese medicine has been gleaned from the *Yellow Emperor's Nei Ching* (a classic text of Chinese internal medicine), which formerly was thought to date from before the year 2000 B.C., but is now thought to be from the second century B.C. The views of the Chinese and the American Indians differ from the natural philosophy of the Western world, but the traditional systems of these widely differing cultures are strikingly similar to those of the West and of other cultures. Like the American Indians, the Chinese use religious, magical, and herbal cures. In addition, Chinese medicine uses acupuncture, ginseng, meditation, and introspective therapy. In contrast to many other cultures, the Chinese have actively attempted to combine their traditional medicine with modern scientific practices.

Choosing a Therapy

Some feel that holistic medicine is a hoax, while others swear by it. Some feel that Western medicine is not correct in its approach to the person, body, and disease. The end result is that there are as many different therapies as there are people, and the one "right" therapy is the protocol that will be picked after looking at many of the treatments available.

The decision to follow any one plan of action should be made with the help of a physician. Many physicians today realize that their patients use alternative medicines and are more than willing to help them explore these options.

Treatments and How They Work

Vaccines

For most people who were born after 1950, there have been few viral diseases that threaten life. The development of vaccines that prevent childhood diseases such as polio, measles, and rubella allowed those who were born in the late '50s and beyond to grow up in a world where there were no killer diseases. For the vast majority of people, the concept of vaccination is nothing new or unusual. Most think that vaccines cure disease and that, between vaccines and antibiotics, a person's being killed by an infection is something that cannot happen. Of course, this idea is far from the truth. Vaccines are the standard treatment for viral infections, but HIV presents a colossal challenge to the development of a vaccine. Understanding this challenge requires an understanding of what a vaccine is and how it works.

Until recently, vaccines were made from naturally occurring viruses or bacteria or from the products of these pathogens. Vaccines may be prepared from live pathogens that have been weakened or attenuated in some way. This technique prevents the pathogen from causing serious disease while still stimulating the immune system to produce antibodies. The antibodies formed against live pathogens last longer; however, the vaccines may not be as safe as ones made from killed organisms. Vaccines made from weakened viruses include those for polio and yellow fever.

The second type of vaccine consists of dead viruses. If the virus can be killed with only a few treatments, it will still stimulate the production of antibodies. While these vaccines are among the safest, the antibodies may not be as numerous as those elicited by live-pathogen vaccines. Diseases for which killed-virus vaccines are used include typhoid fever, rabies, and whooping cough.

A third type of vaccine produces antibodies that fight against the poisons, or toxins, generated by pathogens. These vaccines contain chemically changed toxins and are considered safe and highly effective. The diphtheria and tetanus vaccines are made in this manner.

Finally, some vaccines, like Jenner's vaccine, consist of viral or bacterial particles that do not cause serious disease but resemble their disease-causing counterparts. These impostors can fool the immune system into producing antibodies against both diseases.

The principle of vaccination is to cause the immune system to behave as though the body has contracted a disease. This sets in motion the body's defense system without risking the damage that may be caused by the disease itself. Immunization can be either active or passive.

In active immunization, the components of the vaccine teach the individual's immune system to recognize a specific toxin, virus, or bacterium. Each pathogen, or disease-causing agent, is identified by *antigens*, or marker molecules, on its surface. The immune system has cells called *B lymphocytes* that detect these antigens and respond by manufacturing molecules called *antibodies*. Each antibody is made specifically to attack one type of antigen. The antibody combines with the antigen—like a key fitting a lock—and enables the immune system to destroy it. If the same type of pathogen enters the body again in the future, its antigens will be recognized, specific antibodies will be rapidly manufactured, and the organism that could cause a disease will be destroyed.

The protection against specific diseases conferred by active immunization generally lasts for years. If the antibodies formed after a vaccination decrease significantly over time, the individual can be revaccinated. So-called "booster shots" cause antibodies to be formed more quickly than they are by the first shot.

Passive immunization involves injecting antibodies made by one person or animal into the bloodstream of another. This type of immunization may be used if active immunization is not available, if an individual has already been exposed to a disease and does not have time to manufacture antibodies, or if an individual's own immune system is not working properly. Passive immunization protects an individual for only a few weeks or months.

Other diseases, such as influenza, are caused by organisms that have the ability to change their antigens from time to time. A new influenza vaccine must be prepared each year to protect against the forms of the flu virus that researchers predict will strike the population during the upcoming flu season.

A third category of organisms has the capacity to hide from the immune system. Some members of the herpes virus family, which can cause cold sores, genital sores, shingles, chicken pox, and mononucleosis, live in nerve roots, where they can avoid detection by blood-borne B lymphocytes. The body's immune system cannot distinguish between the nerve root and the pathogen.

Technical problems have also hindered the development of vaccines. Research is expensive. Most of the drugs that are researched do not make it out to the public. It costs millions of dollars to develop a drug through the various testing procedures and finally into manufacture. Vaccines have side effects that can be quite serious for some individuals. Drug companies may be reluctant to produce vaccines because of the threat of lawsuits from those who may be harmed by these side effects. Even many existing vaccines have not been widely used in developing countries because of problems with storing and administering the doses. In some areas of the world, there are still major outbreaks of measles and polio, even now that there are very effective vaccines that can be used to prevent them.

Immune-Bolstering Therapies

Immune boosters attempt to rebuild or stimulate the immune system. These therapies are still in the early experimental stages, and they are not performing as effectively as was hoped. This does not mean, however, that they are not going to be refined in the future. They do offer some benefit to the person receiving them, and they also seem to lack serious side effects that antivirals are known to cause. These drugs are still experimental and are being used only in clinical trials. Those who profess to offer immune-bolstering therapy otherwise are more than likely attempting to con the person seeking help.

Antiviral Therapies

There are two things medicine can offer people who have AIDS, aside from treatment for the opportunistic infections: the experimental immune-bolstering therapies just discussed, and antiviral drugs, a number of which have been developed since HIV was first identified. Antiviral drugs focus on inactivating or holding back the AIDS virus itself. The ones in widest current use are Zidovudine and ddI. In general, these drugs slow the progression of HIV for a period of time, after which the virus mutates and becomes resistant. Antiviral therapies are grouped into two families: the nonnucleoside reverse transcriptase inhibitors (NNRTIs) and the nucleoside-analog reverse transcriptase inhibitors (NARTIs). Nonnucleoside reverse transcriptase inhibitors include such drugs as BI-RG-587, pyridinone, nevrapine, TIBO derivatives, and BHAP compound. These drugs have been shown to inhibit HIV replication in vitro by attacking the reverse transcriptase enzyme, which is the mechanism by which HIV creates a DNA analog with its RNA. When this enzyme is destroyed, the virus cannot transcribe its RNA into DNA and is thus rendered harmless. NNRTI drugs also include zidovudine, ddC, and ddI; there is great debate as to the effectiveness of these drugs. There are some studies that suggest that they do work to limit the amount of HIV in the body, but most studies have confirmed that these drugs currently do not prolong life or prevent HIV infection from progressing to AIDS.

Zidovudine

Zidovudine (previously known as AZT) is used either alone or in combination with zalcitabine (ddC) in the treatment of the infection caused by HIV. Zidovudine is used to slow the progression of disease in patients infected with HIV who have advanced symptoms, early symptoms, or no symptoms at all. This medicine also is used to help prevent pregnant women who have HIV from passing the virus to their babies during pregnancy and at birth.

Zidovudine will not cure or prevent HIV infection or AIDS; however, it helps keep HIV from reproducing and appears to slow the destruction of the immune system, which in turn may help delay the development of problems usually related to AIDS or HIV disease. Zidovudine will not keep a person with HIV from spreading the virus to other people. People who receive this medicine may continue to have the problems usually related to AIDS or HIV disease.

Zidovudine may cause some serious side effects, including bone marrow problems. Symptoms of bone marrow problems include fever and chills, or sore throat, pale skin, and unusual tiredness or weakness. These problems may require blood transfusions or temporary cessation of treatment with zidovudine. The patient's doctor should be consulted if any new health problems or symptoms occur during the administration of zidovudine.

Zidovudine is available only with a doctor's prescription. It is given to people in two basic forms: orally and by injection into the bloodstream.

In deciding to use a medicine, the risks of taking the medicine must be weighed against the good it will do. This is a decision a doctor should make. Doctors need to know any unusual or allergic reaction to zidovudine. They also need to be aware of other allergies to any other substances, such as foods, preservatives, or dyes.

Zidovudine is also known to cross the placenta. Studies in pregnant women have not been completed. However, zidovudine has been shown to decrease the chance of passing HIV to a baby during pregnancy and at birth. Zidovudine has not been shown to cause birth defects in studies in rats and rabbits given this medicine by mouth in doses proportionately many times larger than the human dose.

Zidovudine can cause serious side effects in any person. Therefore, it is especially important that there be open communication concerning the good that this medicine may do as well as the risks of using it. Children must be carefully followed, and frequently seen, by a doctor while taking zidovudine.

Zidovudine has not been studied specifically in older people. This is primarily because of the low incidence of HIV infection in older populations as well as the fact that most clinical trials do not use older people, as the side effects can be very serious and are better tolerated by younger people. Therefore, it is not known whether the drug causes different side effects or problems in the elderly than it does in younger adults.

Although certain medicines should not be used together at all, in other cases two different medicines may be used together even if an interaction might occur. In these cases, a doctor may want to change the dose, or other precautions may be necessary. When zidovudine is being taken, it is especially important that health care professionals know if a person is taking any of the following drugs: amphotericin B by injection (Fungizone), antineoplastics (cancer medicine), antithyroid agents (medicine for overactive thyroid), azathioprine (Imuran), chloramphenicol (Chloromycetin), colchicine, cyclophosphamide (Cytoxan), flucytosine (Ancobon), ganciclovir (Cytovene), interferon (Intron A, Roferon-A), mercaptopurine (Purinethol), methotrexate (Mexate), or pilcamycin (Mithracin).

Many of these medications can cause serious side effects with HIV. Taking AZT while using or receiving these medicines may cause anemia and other blood problems to worsen.

There are also some drugs that will interact with AZT and reduce the effectiveness of the drug; for example, clarithromycin (Biaxin) may decrease bioavailability of AZT in the blood. Conversely, some medications such as probenecid (Benemid) may increase the amount of zidovudine in the blood, increasing the chance of side effects.

This medicine should be taken exactly as directed by a doctor. It should not be taken in higher doses, nor should it be taken more often or for a longer time than a doctor has ordered. Likewise, a person should not discontinue taking this medicine without checking with a doctor. For those using zidovudine syrup, a specially marked spoon or other dispenser to measure each dose accurately should be used, and this spoon should be washed and stored away from other spoons. Taking these precautions will ensure that dosages are relatively uniform. It should also be remembered that the average household teaspoon may not hold the right amount of liquid.

This medicine works best when there is a constant amount in the blood. To help keep the amount constant, doses should not be missed.

Missed Doses. It is sometimes difficult or impossible to take medications at the scheduled time. If a dose of this medicine is missed, it should be taken as soon as possible. However, if it is almost time for the next dose, it is better to skip the missed dose and go back to a regular dosing schedule.

Storing AZT. This medicine, like all medicines, should be stored out of the reach of children. It should be stored away from heat and direct light. It should not be stored in the bathroom, near the kitchen sink, or in other damp places, as heat or moisture may cause the medicine to break down. Outdated medicine or medicine no longer needed should be flushed down a drain.

The Side Effects of AZT. Along with its needed effects, a medication may cause some unwanted effects. Although not all of these side effects may occur, often they need medical attention. A person should record when the side effects take place in relation to when the drug was administered, what was taken with the medication, and the amount of the medication that was taken at the time when the side effects were first noticed. Common side effects are fevers, chills, sore throat, pale skin, and unusual tiredness or weakness. Often, these side effects will go away after the patient has stopped taking the medication, but for some the effects will persist weeks or months after stopping this medicine.

In rare cases, zidovudine may cause abdominal discomfort, confusion, convulsion (seizures), a general feeling of discomfort, loss of appetite, mood or mental changes, muscle tenderness and weakness, and severe nausea. Other side effects may occur that usually do not need medical attention. These may go away during treatment as the body adjusts to the medicine. However, a doctor should be consulted if any of the following side effects continue for a prolonged period of time: headaches (severe), muscle soreness, nausea, trouble sleeping, or any other chronic problem that has been caused by using this medication.

Zalcitabine

Zalcitabine (known as ddC) is used in the treatment of the infection caused by HIV, and is available only with a doctor's prescription, in tablet form.

Zalcitabine, like zidovudine, will not cure or prevent HIV infection or AIDS; however, it helps keep HIV from reproducing and appears to slow the destruction of the immune system, which again may help delay the development of problems usually related to AIDS or HIV disease. As with AZT, zalcitabine will not prevent an infected person from spreading HIV to other people. People who receive this medicine may continue to have other problems usually related to AIDS or HIV disease.

Zalcitabine may cause some serious side effects, including peripheral neuropathy (a problem involving the degeneration of the nerves of the hands and feet). Symptoms of peripheral neuropathy include tingling, burning, numbness, or pain in the hands or feet. Zalcitabine may also cause pancreatitis (inflammation of the pancreas). Symptoms of pancreatitis include stomach pain and nausea.

Zalcitabine has not been studied in pregnant women. How ever, studies in animals have shown that zalcitabine causes birth defects when given in very high doses.

When zalcitabine is being taken, it is especially important that health care professionals know if a person is taking any of the following drugs: azathioprine (Imuran), estrogen (female hormones), alcohol, asparaginase (Elspar), furosemide (Lasix), methyldopa (Aldomet), pentamidine by injection (Pentam, Pentacarinat), sulfonamides (Bactrim, Septra), sulindac (Clinoril), tetracyclines, thiazide diuretics (water pills) (Diuril, Hydrodiuril), or valproic acid (Depakote). These medicines, when used with zalcitabine, may increase the chance of pancreatitis (inflammation of the pancreas).

The use of antacids with zalcitabine may decrease the absorption of zalcitabine; antacids and zalcitabine should not be taken at the same time. Other medical problems that should be considered when using this drug are: alcohol abuse, increased blood triglycerides, or a history of pancreatitis. Those with liver disease should be careful, as zalcitabine may make liver disease worse, especially in patients with a history of alcohol abuse.

The dose of zalcitabine will be different for different patients. The patient should follow the doctor's orders or the directions on the label. The following information stipulates only the average doses: adults and children 13 years of age and older, 0.75 milligram (mg), together with 200 mg of zidovudine, every 8 hours; or 0.75 mg alone every 8 hours. Use and dosage for children up to 12 years of age are to be determined by the doctor. If a dose is missed, it should be taken as soon as possible. However, if it is almost time for the next dose, it is best to skip the missed dose and return to a regular dosing schedule. Double doses should not be taken. This drug should be stored in the same manner as zidovudine.

Didanosine

Didanosine (ddI) is used in the treatment of the infection caused by HIV. This drug may cause some serious side effects, including pancreatitis. Didanosine may also cause peripheral neuropathy. Considerations to be taken into account before using didanosine are discussed below.

Diet. Health care professionals must know if a person who might be given ddI is on any special diet, such as a low sodium (low salt) diet. Didanosine chewable tablets and the oral solution packets contain a large amount of sodium, and this should not be taken by those who have high blood pressure, for example. Also, ddI tablets contain phenylalanine, which must be restricted in patients with phenylketonuria (PKU). This is especially important for young children who have PKU, as neurological problems will result from taking phenylalanine.

Pregnancy. Didanosine crosses the placenta. Studies in pregnant women have not been done. However, ddI has not been shown to cause birth defects or other problems in animal studies. Also, it is not known whether didanosine reduces the chance that a baby born to an HIV-infected mother will also be infected.

Breast Feeding. It is not known whether ddI passes into the breast milk. However, if a baby does not already have the AIDS virus, there is a chance that AIDS could be passed to the baby by breast feeding. Those women who are HIV positive and are thinking about breast feeding should talk to their physicians about this.

It is not known whether ddI causes different side effects or problems in older people. There is no specific information comparing use of ddI in the elderly with use in other age groups.

Didanosine in Combination with Other Medicines. When didanosine is being taken, it is especially important that the health care professional know if any of the following drugs are being taken: alcohol, asparaginase (Elspar), azathioprine (e.g., Imuran), estrogens (female hormones), furosemide (Lasix), sulfonamides (Bactrim, Septra), sulindac (Clinoril), thiazide diuretics (Diuril, Hydrodiuril), valproic acid (Depakote).

Use of the following medications with didanosine may increase the chance of pancreatitis: chloramphenicol (Chloromycetin), cisplatin (Platinol), ethambutol (Myambutol), ethionamide (Trecator-SC), hydralazine (Apresoline), isoniazid (Nydrazid), lithium (Eskalith, Lithobid), nitrous oxide, phenytoin (Dilantin), stavudine (D4T), vincristine (Oncovin), or zalcitabine (HIVID).

Use of the following medicines with didanosine may increase the chance of peripheral neuropathy: ciprofloxacin (Cipro), enoxacin (Penetrax), itraconzole (Sporanox), ketoconazole (Nizoral), lomefloxacin (Maxaquin), norfloxacin (Noroxin), ofloxacin (e.g., Floxin).

Use of the medicines listed below with didanosine may keep these medicines from working properly; these medicines should be taken at least 2 hours before or 2 hours after taking didanosine.

- Dapsone (e.g., Avlosulfon): Use of dapsone with didanosine may increase the chance of peripheral neuropathy; it may also keep dapsone from working properly.
- Nitrofurantoin (e.g., Macrodantin): Use of nitrofurantoin with didanosine may increase the chance of pancreatitis and peripheral neuropathy.
- Tetracyclines (e.g., Achromycin, Minocin): Use of tetracyclines with didanosine may increase the chance of pancreatitis; it may also keep the tetracycline from working properly.

Dosage. For adults and teenagers, the dose is based on body weight. For those who weigh less than 60 kilograms (kg) (132 pounds): 167 milligrams (mg) every 12 hours. For patients weighing 60 kilograms (kg; 132 pounds) or more: 250 mg every 12 hours.

For children, the dose is based on body size and must be determined by a doctor. The usual dose ranges from 31 to 125 mg every 8–12 hours.

If a dose of this medicine is missed, it should be taken as soon as possible. However, if it is almost time for the next dose, the missed dose should be skipped and the regular dosing schedule resumed with the next dose. A double dose should not be taken.

Protease Inhibitors

A new class of AIDS drugs called *protease inhibitors* have recently been discovered. Unlike earlier AIDS therapies, Crixivan, as yet the only one of these drugs to undergo clinical trials, attacks HIV during a later stage in its life cycle. These drugs act to interrupt the production of protease, an enzyme that is crucial to HIV reproduction. Crixivan is not a cure for AIDS, but has had a promising effect on reducing viral level and has also shown CD4 cell recovery. Patients taking Crixivan, in combination with two other AIDS medications, achieved significant reductions in the level of HIV in the bloodstream, according to a new open-label study at the Third Conference on Retroviruses and Opportunistic Infections (January 1996).

Crixivan, when taken with the AIDS medications AZT and ddI, has been shown to reduce virus levels by approximately 99.9% or 1000-fold (2.9 copies/mm^3). Moreover, the level of virus in the bloodstream was reduced to below detectable levels (200 copies/mm^3) in 59% of those who received the drug ($N = 22$) for 5 months. People entered the study with median viral levels of approximately 100,000 copies/mm^3.

These people also experienced significant immune system recovery. On average, people's T-cell counts increased by 90 cells/mm^3. Before taking the medication, most had T-cell counts of 150 cells/mm^3. After 6 months of treatment, patients taking Crixivan alone had a median increase of 85 T cells/mm^3, while patients taking AZT in combination with ddI had a median increase of 30 cells/mm^3.

It appears that this medication is generally well tolerated. No cases of nephrolithiasis (defined as flank pain, blood in the urine, or kidney stones) occurred in the patients in this study. Nephrolithiasis has occurred in some people taking this therapy, however; it has been reported in 2–3% of patients in other Crixivan studies.

Those in clinical trials were encouraged to drink water to maintain hydration, and the vast majority of patients who experienced nephrolithiasis continued on therapy without dose reduction. There were significant drug interactions seen with rifabutin and ketoconazole, which have been managed with dose adjustments.

Summary

There are many different approaches to treating disease. Some approach the treatment of AIDS using alternative forms of medicine; others continue with medical treatments that have been grouped together and termed "Western" medicine. All these therapies have benefits as well as drawbacks.

Those who work with AIDS patients looking for medical assistance should be sure to inform their clients that, in the United States, most health insurance companies compensate only for care that is approved—that is, Western medicine.

The most important aspect of the medical treatment of AIDS is to understand that there is a wide range of treatments from which to choose. Those who are seeking to choose from among these treatments should feel comfortable with their physician. They should be able to ask him questions and get honest answers.

7

The People Who Have AIDS

AIDS affects people from all walks of life, but it touches certain groups more than others—specifically, gay men, minority women, sex trade workers, and those who use injection drugs and share their "works." These groups of people are often hidden from so-called "mainstream" society. When a gay man or woman is depicted on television or in a film, he or she is often the object of jokes or ridicule, a so-called "safe" reflexive reaction from a society in which these people are overlooked. The results of this type of thought paradigm are significant; those who have HIV or AIDS historically have been denied respect or equality, and the failure to accord them these decencies is one of the factors that has made HIV so prevalent in the United States. It was once thought that HIV was not going to affect the mainstream population; indeed, it was rarely even mentioned that, to a virus, there is no such thing as a "mainstream population." As a society, we defined AIDS as a disease that hurt only those who "did something to deserve it." It was this myopic perspective that acted as a catalyst for the rapid spread of HIV in the United States; those with HIV were labeled as "fringe" groups and thought to exist in a vacuum. The concept of "fringe groups" is a misnomer, and our allowing this to continue will only continue to take energy and resources from a stressed system that attempts to help those who have HIV and those who work to prevent its further spread. To change the concept of fringe groups means to change the ideas that exist in people's minds concerning the populations in which AIDS is endemic.

Gay Men

The term *homosexuality* (derived from the Greek *homo* meaning "same"—*not* from the Latin *homo*, meaning "man") was coined in 1869 by Karl Maria Kerbeny, who wrote a paper against Prussia's antihomosexual laws. The term *gay* became prevalent in the late 1960s and now usually refers to homosexual men; the term *lesbian* (derived from the Greek island of Lesbos, home of the reputed homosexual band surrounding Sappho, a 6th-century B.C. poet) refers to homosexual women.

Historically, this group has not been visible to the general population except in the rare cases of a movie that vilified them ("Silence of the Lambs") or, recently, one that portrays them as flamboyant, artsy, acid-tongued men who always have great taste ("The Birdcage"). What is missing in these films is a real portrayal of gay men as ordinary people. Moreover, there is little discussion concerning the struggles that homosexuals have faced throughout history and the fact that AIDS is *not* what started the "gay rights" movement. This is an important aspect, in that gay rights and AIDS are not the same issue, but they are connected.

The History of the Gay Community Movement

By the 1920s, many urban centers had developed "gay" culture, but societal prejudice kept this small segment of society well hidden. The development of large urban centers created a new social dynamic. A person could now live in anonymity. Families changed; young adults left home to find jobs, and it was acceptable to live alone. Having a private life allowed individuals to acknowledge their sexuality, and soon there were groups collectively identifying themselves as being attracted to people of the same gender.

In the 1940s, urban populations exploded. People were moving into cities to find jobs and join the war effort, and in this influx of people there were, of course, gays and lesbians. It was also noted in the 1940s that the first gay bars were opened in New York City, and social networks developed. This increased the visibility of gays and acted as a catalyst for public policy that subjugated homosexuals. An example of this was an order from then-President Dwight D. Eisenhower that barred gays and lesbians from all government jobs and military service. On local government levels, vice squads made efforts to harass gay citizens who went to gay bars, often arresting dozens of men and women.

The actions that the government took to repress homosexual activity sparked the "gay rights" movement. In November 1950, the Mattachine Society was formed by Harry Hay and Chuck Rowland in Los Angeles. In 1955, a lesbian group, the Daughters of Bilitis, founded by Del Martin and Phyllis Lyon, joined forces with the Mattachine Society. The organization remained small but did establish chapters in other cities and published information about the gay movement.

It was during the 1960s that the gay rights movement gathered more strength in advocating for equality and basic civil rights. In Washington, the activists Franklin Kameny and Barbara Gittings protested discriminatory government employment policies. In San Francisco, protesters targeted the local police to end harassment.

The protest efforts culminated on June 27, 1969, when the New York City Police Department raided a well-known Greenwich Village gay bar, the Stonewall Inn. In a totally unanticipated response to the police raid, the patrons fought back, joined by many sympathetic heterosexual people in the crowd. The three nights of rioting changed a small local movement into the national spotlight. The first year after the riots, 5000 men and women marched in New York City to commemorate what was to many the birth of the gay rights movement. By 1973, there were over 750 gay organizations across the United States.

The gay rights movement was then and is now a struggle for equality. It began as a protest against the prejudice that gay men and women faced across the country. It was not, and still is not, a fight for special or different rights, and should not be categorized as anything other than a movement to end oppression. Gays and lesbians are forced to live with the fear of losing jobs, homes, and possibly their lives. Before the movement to secure gay rights in the 1960s, the violence that gays and lesbians were subjected to was not acknowledged. During World War II, the Nazis ferreted out gays and lesbians, imprisoned them in concentration camps, and labeled them with an inverted pink triangle. Like the Jews, gays and lesbians were experimented on, tortured, and killed. Unlike many of the groups victimized by the Nazis, gays were not acknowledged in the Nuremburg Trials. Later, when the United Nations wrote the Declaration of Human Rights, crimes committed against gays and lesbians were not addressed. To survive in this world, gays and lesbians were forced to start seeking civil equality.

As the gay and lesbian movement continued to gather momentum and power in the 1960s and 1970s, there was, not surprisingly, a backlash from conservatives. In 1977, the public attack on gays and lesbians was fueled by singer Anita Bryant, who was trying to repeal a gay rights ordinance in Dade County, Florida. The ordinance was intended to legislate equal treatment for housing, jobs, and partnerships. This type of proposal does not give gays and lesbians more rights than other people, but merely requires that people keep personal prejudices out of the decision-making process that affects a person's ability to secure a job, loan, or place to live.

It can only be upsetting to be painted as a so-called pervert to the world. What is it like for a gay or lesbian person to turn on the news and listen to people talk about their peers the way they do in our society? What must it be like to be vilified by major institutions, such as the military, for beliefs and motivations that neither hurt nor destroy? This is an inevitable part of the gay or lesbian experience in the United States. Understanding a person and his experience is a fundamental key to empathy. In all health care settings, it is acknowledged that good care means knowing the client. For family members, learning about gay rights is often a sign of support and can open up important lines of communication. Many people are shocked to learn about the plight of gays and lesbians, as they are not aware of the legislative, political, and religious policies that discriminate, nor are they aware of how these institutions cause discrimination.

Case Study 7.1

"My son was diagnosed with AIDS in 1990 and died in July of 1991. He had moved away to school and became involved in the gay rights movement. He came out of the closet and then told us, his father and I, what the gay rights movement was all about. At the time, I was so ashamed of my son's homosexuality that I could not even talk about it, let alone gay rights.

"After Adam told us that he was gay, it was as if everything I heard from that point on was about gays. On TV, the radio, newspapers, out in public, it seemed that all I heard about was gays. I was so tired of listening to gays and their needs for rights. I was playing bridge with a group of women and the topic came up. It was so clear, as I was listening to this woman rant on about gays, that what I was hearing all the time was not gays demanding rights, but rather people complaining about gays. I asked this woman what her beef was with the gays, and she looked at me and told me with authority that they were evil, and against the natural law. I asked her why she thought this, and she had no answer, but asked me what this was all about. I guess she thought that I should have deferred to her judgments. At first I said nothing because I did not want to talk about Adam's personal business, but as I sat there I knew better—I was keeping my mouth shut because I was ashamed of Adam. I have never felt such self-loathing before in my life. I let a woman tell me to my face that my smart, charming son was evil, and said nothing. There was nowhere to hide when this realization hit. I never said anything to that woman, but I started attending Parents and Friends of Lesbians and Gays, and researching gay rights and the oppression and violence that they endure on a daily basis.

"My son suffered with AIDS. His upper palate was destroyed by cancer. He lost fifty pounds. He lost his job. He lost so much, and the only thing that gives me comfort today is that he never had to feel, that afternoon at bridge, that he was going through his life without the support of his family. Any person who can think or read should be more aware of what gays and lesbians have to suffer in this world. I once wished desperately that my son was heterosexual. Then I got to know him, as a person, and this required that I accept his sexuality. Then I started to really understand his motivations and experiences and began to see that my son was a brave man like no other. I fell in love with this man all over again, like I did the day that I first held him in the hospital.

"Then this disease took my baby, my friend, and hero. There are no words that describe my loss nor ones that can heal it. I think about what people say about gays and lesbians and it is evil, it is hateful, it is hurtful, it should not be tolerated! Who would ever think that I would be a gay rights activist? Some might say that it is ironic. I think it a moral duty."

MARY, 67, mother and activist

Religion and Homosexuality

Many religious groups declare homosexuality immoral and sinful, causing problems when they want to establish government policy based on religious doctrine. These objections to homosexuality are not grounded or supported by statistics that suggest that homosexuality is any more "abnormal" than heterosexuality is normal. Often, the objections are based on interpretations of biblical scripture. The Bible, though, concentrates very little on homosexuality or on the condemnation of it. The Bible contains over 30,000 verses, of which only 9 passages refer to, or can be interpreted as having relevance to, homosexuality. Four verses, Deuteronomy 23:17, I Kings 14:24, I Kings 22:46, and II Kings 23:7, forbid prostitution for both men and women. Two passages and one verse in the Gospel of St. Paul may be interpreted as calling homosexuality wrong: Romans 1:25–2:1, I Corinthians 6:9–11, and I Timothy 1:10. What is often missed in examining these passages, however, is the context in which they were written. This was a time when Roman culture was being challenged by the ideology of the Judeo-Christian leaders. The teachings of Jesus proclaimed the value of spiritual development opposing the pleasures of the flesh. Paul's writings, given this information, can better be seen as propaganda to discredit the Roman norms, rather than a divinely approved attack on homosexuality. The fact that there is no theological objection to homosexuality in the New Testament lends more evidence to the view that the Old Testament's writings represented opposition to the Roman lifestyle in general.

Possibly the most damning biblical passages are Leviticus 18:19–23 and Leviticus 20:10–16, which do forbid homosexuality, yet are also part of the "Holiness Code," which also bans eating raw meat, sexual relations while menstruating, tattooing, planting two different crops in the same field, and wearing clothes that are made of different types of yarn. Clearly, the demands of the Holiness Code were expected not to be followed in everyday life, except, apparently, in their application to gay men and women.

What most fail to see is that even if the Bible does in fact state that homosexual unions are wrong, this does not mean that society should be forced to bend to the norms prescribed by one religion.

Most organized religions have a philosophy concerning homosexuality (see Table 7.1). Some of the more common religious groups classify homosexuality as a sin and ban its practice. When a religious group lobbies against homosexuality in a political

Table 7.1. Religions and Their Policies Concerning
Homosexuality

Religion	Philosophy on homosexuality
United Methodist	1, 3
Mormons	2, 4
Baptists	1, 4
Episcopal	1, 3
Lutherans	1, 4
Muslims	2, 4
Orthodox Jews	4
Reform and Reconstructionist Jews	1, 3
Catholics	1, 4
Buddhists	1, 3

1 = Gays and lesbians can join religious group; 2 = Gays and lesbians not welcome; 3 = Faith does not consider homosexuality a sin; 4 = Faith does consider homosexuality a sin

arena, it affects society's attitudes toward gays and lesbians. These attitudes in turn affect the treatment gays and lesbians receive. Those in the helping professions should examine some of the more restrictive policies and understand the efforts that are being made to subjugate gays and lesbians.

Case Study 7.2

"A friend's son was diagnosed with AIDS and died. He was living in San Francisco, and his mother did not even tell me that he was sick until she had to fly out when he was dying. I was heartbroken by her isolation and pain. When she told me what was going on, I was just devastated, and I decided that I wanted to help in some way in the AIDS crisis. I went to my church, I am a Roman Catholic, and investigated to see if there were any efforts that were being made to help people who had AIDS, and there were plenty. I started to go once every two weeks to a home for men and women who have AIDS.

"I was sitting with a young man [Eric] who was blind because of the disease, and he was asking me why I was doing this, coming in and helping out. I told him that I was a Catholic and felt that it was my duty as a Christian to help people when they need it. He asked me if I believed in what the Catholic faith said about gays, and I told him that I believed in the teachings of the church—I didn't know at the time what the church was saying about gays.

"He was pretty cool to me after this exchange, and I did not know why. I used to come in and read *People* magazine to him, and we would laugh about the articles, but all of this stopped. I was confused and asked the volunteer coordinator about it. She told me to go to Eric and ask him if there was something troubling him. I went to his room and sat down on the chair and asked him if he was okay, and he said that he was fine. He was not mean, but very distant. I asked him if he was angry with me, and he said that he was angry with people who discriminate and label him a sinner. I was so shocked, because I do not think that I am a bigot. I told him that I do not discriminate and he explained to me the policies of the church on homosexuality.

"To be honest, I did not believe him, and I did not think that the Catholic Church took such a stand. I asked my priest about it and he confirmed what Eric had told me. I felt so badly, just so badly. Like that suffering man needed to be told by his reader that I thought his life and relationships were an abomination! I was thrilled that I had the opportunity to tell Eric that I was a Catholic who rejected the narrow teachings of my faith in this regard. It opened up a dialogue between us about faith and death and what happens to us all. What an important issue that faith is for the sick; it is vile that so many faiths push their hate to exclude these men and women. No God wants this! That's the faith: knowing that no God would want such hate even if the leaders of the church said it was correct. Even Jesus rejected the teachings of the church leaders of his day."

MARY, 57, *volunteer*

There are some groups that more than others seem to have a need not only to call out against homosexuals, but also to limit what they can do in society. In 1990, the National Conference of Catholic Bishops provided a document on human behavior that labeled homosexual behavior evil. A Bishop from St. Louis, Edward O'Donnel, said that the "tendency or the orientation is a disorder, but the person is not an evil person." In 1992, the Vatican ordered American bishops to preach against any legislation that allows gays to serve in the armed forces, work in child care, teach in schools, have a coaching position, or adopt children. So, although the church claims to value homosexuals in the same way it values all other human beings, the message heard by the 52 million Catholics of the United States is that there is something wrong with gay men and lesbians, and that they should be treated accordingly.

The Catholic Church is not the only group that openly attacks homosexuality. The Traditional Values Coalition, based in Anaheim, California, attempted to make it illegal to enact laws that protect gays and lesbians from discrimination. Pat Robertson, who heads the 700 Club and was the founder of the Christian Coalition, openly states that homosexuals recruit young people for sexual acts, suggesting that gay men are pedophiles, even though statistics show that child molesters are heterosexuals in over 95% of all sexual abuse cases. Then there is the Rev. Jerry Faldwell, who stated that Americans "must awaken to their [homosexuals'] wicked agenda for America."

The point that gays and lesbians are condemned by society's most "spiritual" arbiters, who declare what is right and wrong, is one to remember when trying to understand the gay experience.

Hate Crimes

A hate crime is defined by a perpetrator's perception that the victim belongs to a certain group. This means that any person who appears to belong to a group in the eyes of the perpetrator is at risk for being a victim of hate crimes. Proportionally, the number of hate crimes against gays and lesbians is higher than crimes against other groups known to be at risk for hate crimes. In a study conducted by the National Gay and Lesbian Task Force (NGLTF 1984) that spoke with 2074 gay and lesbian people, 19% said they had been punched, kicked, or beaten at least once in their lives because they were homosexual; 44% stated that they had been threatened with physical violence; 94% reported that they had experienced some type of threat, such as being spit on or called epithets; and 83% said that they felt there was a good chance that they would experience physical violence in the future because of their sexuality.

The hatred that compels someone to attack another must be overwhelming for the aggressor, but for the victim it is frightening and possibly deadly.

Case Study 7.3

"It started when I was in high school. Oh, wait ... maybe it was before then, I don't remember. I just remember it getting unbearable in the ninth grade. The older boys seemed to sense that I was different. I don't know what it was or why I was so important to them, but they were always picking on me. It started out as name calling, but they would do it like in front of the whole gym class, or on the bus. Then they started to get more aggressive. They would come up to me at my locker and push me, or punch my arm. Teachers would pretend when they saw this shit that it was all just fun and games, but it was not, and they knew it. These guys were the jocks and everyone liked them. I don't know why. They were mean, cruel, and violent. One Saturday, it was in the summer and I was walking home from the public pool, and these two guys who were real jerks were walking down the street, and I knew they would do something, and they did. They punched me in the nose and broke it. I started to cry and they said, 'A cry baby and a faggot,' and I was 'lucky they didn't kick my ass.'"

CORY, 25, *social worker*
Coordinator of Gay and Lesbian Youth Project

Imagine that after an episode of violence such as this, society's attention were to be directed, not at the violent behavior, but at the person who was the recipient of the violence. Such a change of viewpoint is a powerful technique and can lend insight into the way society assesses blame where gay men and women are involved. It is not hard to see the disdain that society has for gay people, nor is it hard to see how this feeling might be extrapolated into other areas that might be seen as a gay issue, such as AIDS.

The hatred of homosexuals has a direct effect on the way society treats those with AIDS. AIDS symbolizes the power of the gay rights movement; not since the Stonewall riots has the gay community had such a sweeping effect on policy, politics, and health care. But it was not the fact that these activists changed policy; it was that they voiced their opinion in a world where they were not permitted to speak. Gay men and women were things to poke fun at, mimic, and label as sick, perverted predators. Gays did not rally against many of the pejorative norms that excluded them from serving in the military, benefiting from legal partnerships, and many other advantages afforded to heterosexuals. But then came AIDS, and those affected most by the virus came together to try to find some relief. Actions taken to support and help those with the disease were viewed as a threat by those who for decades tried to keep homosexuals in the shadows. While AIDS has pushed the "gay agenda," and facilitated unity, the slights experienced by gays and their desires to be treated as equal were always there.

It was this societal disdain of homosexuality that kept President Reagan from dealing with the disease for years and that kept the public from demanding that he do so. The administration stated that AIDS was not going to be an issue for the heterosexual population. This view was not widely challenged, although it must have been clear that a sexually transmitted disease was not going to be contained by silence alone. The physical process of dying from AIDS is awful, but it must be excruciating to be attacked with hateful policies, blame, and jeers as one is dying. Gay men responded to this treatment with venom, and they used the media in order to be widely seen—and they *were* seen—in a sympathetic light. The actions of ACT UP were often met with hostility and disgust in middle America; yet, as the AIDS crisis became larger, so did the actions of groups such as ACT UP.

Case Study 7.4

"I was coming home from shopping with my sister on Saturday afternoon. We had been at the mall and decided to stop at McDonald's for lunch. We were waiting in line, the place was very crowded, and I saw a group of men who were in the next line over and were slightly ahead of me and my sister. One of the men was wearing a T-shirt that said, 'Silly Faggot, Dicks Are for Chicks.' It was a parody of the rabbit from the Trix cereal commercials. It was the most offensive display of hate and intolerance that I had seen, but that was not the worst part. The place was packed and not one person said a word about the shirt. I wonder if it were a shirt about blacks or a slam on Christianity, I wonder if a person would feel comfortable enough to wear such a shirt, and if people would be comfortable in seeing such a shirt in McDonald's. It was so hurtful, not only to me, but I know it hurts those who care about me, and do not want to see me subjected to this. It was just so humiliating, to have the part of you that is so intimate, that connects you to another person in a special way, made fun of in such a way. The shirt really got me, it was so unnecessary."

JAMES, 29, *graduate student*

The impact of hate on the lives of gay people is real. The statistics collected by the United States Department of Justice conclude that hate crimes against homosexuals are increasing, and the incidence of these crimes is underreported. These crimes cause a host of reactions that affect the way gay people are viewed by both themselves and others, and this has an effect on the treatment they receive.

Information for Parents of Gay Men

It is not unusual for parents to learn simultaneously that their son has AIDS and that he is homosexual. Both pieces of information are overwhelming; they force parents to confront fear and anxiety about the precarious health of their child, and, as well, challenge their belief systems about sexuality.

Parents are not socialized to think about the death of their children; the rule is that children survive their parents, not the reverse. A parent's immediate desire is to intervene in the process that is causing such harm. For the parent who learns that his or her child has AIDS, the usual avenues to protect and intervene are denied and cause frustration. Often a dichotomous emotional reaction arises whereby the parent wants to destroy or reject that which he feels is the root of the cause: "If the child were not gay, he would not have AIDS and he would not be dying." The individual is unable to separate himself from his sexuality, and as a result the individual is rejected.

Case Study 7.5

"Gary had moved to New York and had been living there for ten years. We thought that we were close to him, thought that we knew about his life. When he would come home he would talk about girlfriends and being involved in projects at work, and we just thought that he was a regular kind of guy.

"We got a call one night from our daughter telling us that Gary was in the hospital with pneumonia. We flew out to New York the next day and were told at the hospital that Gary had AIDS. We went into his room and he was so sick. We were there for about an hour when his *friend*, Mike, came in. We had no idea until this moment that he was gay; it was as if the man that we knew as our son no longer existed. Gary was released from the hospital after about a week.

"The night before we were to fly home we all went to his house. It was difficult because we were not sure how to act, and part of me was so mad that he would lie to us and not tell us about his life. When I asked him why he kept this secret he said that he was scared to tell us about his sexuality, because both his father and I had made comments about gays before that he said led him to believe that we did not accept this lifestyle. I told him that it was silly, that he was our son and that we loved him no matter what. He did not really accept this, and went on about how we said these things and it was not his responsibility to explore how much we would tolerate, that he was not willing to risk his family over the issue. I started to cry after a while, because I was sad that he was sick, because I was not going to see his babies, that I was not going to see him married. And then he went wild screaming that it was our fault for allowing the world to treat people this way. He was so sick and this was so taxing for him.

"Like a lot of things that families do, I got mad and started to scream back and then it all hit me that my baby was dying, and I lost it. We spent a lot of time together before he died, and both his father and I were grateful that we both got to share more of his life. I used to think when I first found out that it might be embarrassing to tell people that Gary had AIDS, then I thought that I did not have to tell people. Now I think that there is nothing worse than his death. How he died is irrelevant."

GEORGIA, 67, mother

As seen in this case study, parents make an assumption that their children are heterosexual, and from this assumption comes the expectation of a "traditional family," including a spouse and children. This is part of society's expectation of an individual as he ages. Successful older people have sons-in-law and daughters-in-law and grandchildren. Their roles change from being parents to being grandparents. When a person declares himself gay, parents see this disclosure as a threat to the roles that they are supposed to have as they grow older. This loss needs to be addressed and validated. Often, the difficulty of "coming out" is so great for the gay individual that the sense of loss felt by other members in the family system is not sufficiently acknowledged. To ignore this reaction does nothing but add to the feelings of isolation, disappointment, and resentment. Failure to address these feelings compromises the parents' ability to appreciate the child in a comprehensive and contextualized manner—that is, as a gay person. This is vitally important when AIDS is a part of the equation. The goal for the family is often a simple one: Open up the communication channels so that there can be effective communication before the disease interferes with the functioning of the affected individual. Allowing the family to accept homosexuality and HIV as two issues that have some relationship to each other, and helping them to develop internal support structures to deal with each issue in a safe forum without villainizing the individual in the process is a vital aspect of support.

Gay Spouses

The term "spouse" has an implication of marriage, which is a term that applies to the institution of the committed legal relationship between a man and a woman. This legal status is not accorded to gay people in most states, so the term "gay spouse" has to be one that is self-defined. Is there a length of time that makes a gay relationship "committed," and is a time less than that considered dating? Is there a shared home? What is this claim that they are committed? These are often the questions asked, and while the same questions can be applied to heterosexual relationships, the term is more subjective for gays and lesbians because there are no regulations imposed. The gay spouse is, however, referred to as such or, in such a way, that one could infer that the relationship is special and significant, that the partner is a spouse in an emotional sense.

The spouse of a person who has AIDS is in need of support, which is often not given. Aside from the benefits denied to gay spouses, there is a general lack of sympathy extended to them as they face the death of a partner.

Case Study 7.6

"Mark was diagnosed with AIDS after we had been together for four years. It was a shock to both of us, as neither one of us was promiscuous. When he got sick, it was really hard for me. I had to pay the bills on my paycheck, make sure that the house was being kept up, that he got to the doctor, that he just got out of the house. The whole time I was doing this, I was losing the person that I really loved. Not only was I losing the person that I loved, but I was watching this man who was so active, so much fun, have the life sucked out of him, and it was brutal.

"There were things that people would do for me that I really did appreciate, but these were groups of volunteers, not his family or mine. There were times, too, that I wanted family, not strangers, coming in and helping. I had to be nice to the volunteers, and there were times when I did not want to be nice. I wanted to be mean, I wanted to tear things apart, but I didn't because they were *visiting nurses* and respite workers. When his family or mine would come, it was like they were coming over for lunch or something and I had to be the host for them. I mean, I do not think that they really got it that I was losing something that was so dear to me that I could not grasp the extent of my loss. They were unable to see that my loss was real because the person I loved more than anything didn't have a uterus."

CRAIG, 36, attorney

There is also the guilt that many survivors feel about surviving their lovers. Many times both people are HIV-positive, and the survivor sees clearly the isolation and pain that he will face after seeing his partner's experience. The difference in this case is that the person he depends on will not be there for his dying process. The structures that exist for survivors, specifically, extended family (meaning in-laws or their equivalent), are often gone when one spouse dies, leaving the other feeling both alone and rejected. The solution to such isolation and subjugation is not always available, and often the remedy is to get the surviving spouse to a human services agency where support can be found.

Exercises

Many of the issues that have been brought up can be addressed, though not necessarily resolved, by looking at the values that individuals might hold concerning homosexuality. The following questions are designed to help identify thoughts and value judgments:

1. What are the messages that I have heard about gays and lesbians from my religion?

2. What feelings are generated when I hear the words "gay" and "lesbian"?
3. What is my reaction to jokes that portray gay and lesbian people in derogatory terms?
4. Have I heard about bias-related crimes targeted at gay people?
5. Have I ever been the target of bias-related behavior such as being the butt of ethnic jokes?
6. Are the feelings that I have when this happens (question 5) similar to the feelings that gays and lesbians have when they experience these jokes?
7. How are gays and lesbians portrayed in the movies and TV programs that I watch? Are these accurate portrayals?
8. Do I use such terms as "faggot," "homo," and "dyke" to describe homosexuals?
9. How would I feel if the people who moved next door to me were homosexual? What might these feelings be if the people were, say, black? Hispanic? Asian? Protestant?
10. Do I know any gay people?
11. Do I socialize with people from different racial groups?
12. If I were made aware that there were bias-related crimes in my community, what, if anything, would I do about it?
13. What are the procedures in my workplace to deal with diversity?
14. How would I feel if my child were gay?
15. How would I feel if my brother or sister were gay?
16. What might my reaction be if a person of the same gender asked me out on a date?
17. Should gay people be allowed in the military?
18. How would I feel if my child's teacher were a gay person?
19. Do I support legislation that restricts gay people's rights?
20. How might I feel if I were to see a gay couple holding hands?
21. Should gay people be able to get married and receive the same benefits that married heterosexual couples receive?
22. How might I feel if I had to keep my personal life secret?

23. What do I think about politicians using gay and lesbians as topics for grandstanding?
24. Can I relate to the gay person who has lost a loved one to AIDS, and do I think he or she has the same feelings as a heterosexual person who has lost a spouse?
25. Do I ever take actions to help gay people receive better treatment in society?

These questions are not meant to do anything but make a person think about the way homosexuality is perceived and the reactions that these perceptions might cause. There are no right or wrong answers. It is a good idea to review them periodically to monitor how viewpoints and values change over time and with experience.

Injection Drug Users

The greatest number of AIDS cases in the United States next to gay men are seen in people who use injection drugs. This population is the most difficult to reach and the most difficult to treat. The reasons this group is so difficult to reach have to do with the drug use and the addictive behaviors that continue to place the people in this population at risk. Understanding addiction and its symptoms is key to providing viable intervention in this population.

Addiction as a Disease

Addiction can be looked at as a disease because it has symptoms and its outcome can be predicted. There are stages, and there are treatments available for those who are afflicted.

Addiction is simply the point at which a person is dependent upon a substance in order to function. At first, the person who uses a substance feels good about the experience, not seeing himself as a potential addict, but simply as a person who is experimenting with the substance. The difference is that the person who is not an addict does not obsess about the substance. The addict person does not have these feelings. Eventually, the substance causes a dependence, and the person reaches a point at which he needs the drug, both physically and mentally.

Dependence

Dependence is difficult to define, in that there are people who think they are dependent but are not and those who think they are not but are. There are people who feel they are *physiologically* dependent and those who feel they are *psychologically* dependent. In order to understand the problems that people claim they have or, conversely, deny having, the following terms and definitions concerning substance abuse are used:

Dependence is defined in clinical terms as the pattern of use that leads to impairment in social, professional, or physical functioning. This impairment must occur over the course of 6 months in order for a person to be clinically dependent.

Tolerance is the increased need for a substance in order to get the same feeling that was once experienced with the use of a smaller amount. It is also seen when there is less effect on a person who uses the same amount over time. The following case study illustrates this concept:

Case Study 7.7

"I was drinking since I was 16 years old. At first, I started drinking beers with a few of my friends in the woods behind my mother's house. We all would drink and get smashed, then we would go home. It was really no big deal except that I was always wanting to drink more. I mean, right from the start I was more into it than the rest of the people who I was drinking with. By the time I was 21 in college, I was able to hold my booze. I thought that this was a cool thing, but the fact was that I was able to drink more because I was so used to drinking a lot. It took a lot for me to feel really out of control."

DAREN, 24, *recovering alcoholic*

This case study illustrates increased tolerance. The person reported feeling that he was not able to achieve the same effect as he once had when using a smaller amount of the substance.

As a person becomes more involved with substance abuse, he uses more of the substance than intended. This reflects the increased need for the substance as well as the inability to control the use. A person who is addicted to alcohol might want to go out and have a beer at happy hour, but ends up drinking until 3 o'clock in the morning and gets drunk, even though he intended to have only one drink.

The addicted person usually begins to understand that he is using more of the substance than is desirable and in reaction tries to "cut down" on his use. Often, the person will try to cut down only to find that he is not able to do so. There are often consequences to the behaviors associated with drug abuse. Often, the person will not make it to work, school, or important family functions. The importance of social structures becomes less while, at the same time, the person spends more time trying to set up structures that enable him to use the substance. Such activity might be looking for drugs or seeking out social functions that allow for drug use.

The person who is using drugs to the point of being classified as addicted will most likely realize that he is using drugs to an extent he knows is not healthy or desirable, but ultimately continue to use drugs despite this knowledge.

Finally, a person addicted to substances is likely to experience withdrawal symptoms when the intake is interrupted. Withdrawal usually elicits feelings of agitation, cravings for the substance, and severe mood swings. In many cases, a person will need medical intervention in order to make it through the physical withdrawal. This is a very serious problem and can be fatal. Detoxifying a person who is physically addicted to substances should not be tried without the assistance of a medical doctor.

Addiction and HIV

The problems that exist for the person who is HIV-positive and addicted to substances are many. It is often assumed that the main problem associated with HIV and addiction is the relationship between the use of intravenous needles and HIV transmission. This, however, is not all that needs to be looked at.

Addiction, be it to heroin, alcohol, or any other drug, puts people in a position where they are not able to protect themselves from HIV infection.

Case Study 7.8

"I was not into drugs, I was a drinker. I would go out and get hammered all the time. I started to drink when I was in high school. I always got wasted, and by the time I was in college things were out of control. But I was in a frat and people just thought that I was a real partyer. By the time I graduated, I knew that I was an alcoholic.

"Three years after I got out of college, I was arrested on a DWI charge. I went into treatment and finally stopped using booze. I got tested for HIV and it came out positive. I was really upset, naturally. I know that I got the virus because I was not in control of myself because of the addiction."

JACK, 28

This case study illustrates clearly that all people who are addicted to substances stand a significant risk for HIV infection because of the lack of control that addiction brings to a person's life.

All people who work in the field of addiction treatment should be aware of the significant risk that exists in this population. Many people who enter treatment centers have histories of sexual promiscuity and have shown poor judgment (a hallmark of addiction). All such people, then, should be aware that they need to be tested. Many who work in the treatment field believe that people who are being treated for addiction need to deal with their addiction as the primary issue and not concern themselves with the possibility of being infected with HIV. While this approach makes sense, there does come a point when the person needs to know for a variety of reasons. Obviously, a person who is going to engage in sex needs to know his HIV status, but there are other reasons as well. A person who is addicted often has a fear of HIV. In a treatment facility, there are usually a few patients who are aware that they are HIV-positive, and thus there is often talk about the virus in these settings. Often, the anxiety associated with not knowing one's HIV status is such that it makes the person want to escape, and the way an addict escapes is to get high, be it on alcohol, cocaine, or other substance.

How Drugs Are Used

A needle is used to inject a drug into a vein. Addicts refer to the equipment that is used to facilitate drug use as "works," which consists of the following:

Cooker: This is usually a spoon that is used to hold the drug so that it can be melted into a liquid form. The substance is placed in the spoon as a solid. A flame is held beneath the spoon to melt the substance.

Cotton: Usually a ball, it is used as a filler between the needle and the liquid in the spoon to catch impurities that may not have melted.

Plunger: This is the apparatus that holds the fluid and forces it through the needle.

There are other implements that might be used in administering the drug; however, these are the implements that can transmit the virus from one person to another.

When a person uses IV drugs, he wants to inject the drug into a vein, not into tissue. To ensure that he has hit a vein, he draws back on the plunger so that it fills with blood; this way, he knows that he has the needle in the "right place." This process, called "booting," contaminates the needle, syringe, cooker, filter, and plunger. If another person uses the equipment, he is at risk for infection.

Intervention

There are two ways to intervene in the transmission of the virus: Stop the addiction and educate the person in ways of protecting himself from infection, or of protecting others from infection if he is infected with the virus. The other approach is to help those who are using substances to do so with a reduced risk of harm.

Stopping a person from using substances is a difficult endeavor, and while it is certainly the healthiest and safest way to deal with HIV infection and transmission, it is also the most unlikely way of stopping the transmission of the virus. The disease of addiction is all about being addicted, and people do not stop using drugs simply because there is the threat of disease. After all, the problem with using drugs is that they are harmful. The nature of addiction is such that the person who is using does not have the ability to look out for his best interests. In light of this, there needs to be great care in helping the person who is addicted to reduce the harm while using drugs. In treatment centers, there is often the idea that successful treatment means the end of drug use. HIV challenges this philosophy in that successful treatment must now incorporate the ideas of harm reduction, for the sake not only of the client, but also of the public. Whereas once the professional in the addiction treatment field might have thought there was nothing one could do while the client was still actively abusing drugs, now there are things the professional can do for the active addict.

Harm-Reduction Techniques

In order to stop the spread of the virus in an IDU (injection drug user), there need to be education and programs. While not popular, needle exchange programs do work. This community-based program works by providing needles to those who are willing to exchange their old ones for clean new needles. Programs that incorporate needle exchange are often criticized for "appeasing" the drug addict, instead of prosecuting him. The confusion that arises is complicated by the fact that addiction is a state that the addict seeks at all cost to maintain, and society's response is not a medical approach, but rather one that comes from the criminal justice system. Pounded into the heads of most people is the concept that drug addicts are lazy and demented and that their state is mediated more by their sloth than by disease. The addict's inability to change might have something to do with being treated like a criminal for something that is inherently medical. The prejudice is so profound that programs such as needle exchanges are banned, leaving the addicted person with services that are totally inadequate to deal with a virus like HIV. Sadly, the responses to the needs of this population are similar to the ones that were directed at gay men years ago. The public is largely blind to the facts: AIDS is up in the United States, the presence of an IDU is one of the greatest cofactors in the development of pediatric AIDS cases, and the spread of HIV into the heterosexual population is often the result of women having sex with an IDU. The result is that the HIV prevention programs struggle in this population at a time when more drastic measures are needed to increase compliance.

The most effective way to reduce the risk of HIV infection in an active drug user is to tell him how he can use drugs and at the same time make drug use safer, in terms of spreading HIV to others.

The first goal that should be employed is to stress to the client who is using IV drugs not to share "shooting" equipment. If needles are not shared, then there is no risk that an IV drug user will spread the virus to another user. If people must share needles, or use needles that are not still wrapped in sterile packages, the needles must be cleaned.

Cleaning "works" is accomplished by soaking all parts in a water–bleach solution, 1 part water to 20 parts chlorine bleach. The solution should be drawn all the way up into the syringe so that the chamber is filled with the solution and should then be evacuated. This process should then be repeated. All of the works, including the cooker, need to be thoroughly cleaned in the bleach solution. The cotton that is used as a filter should never be shared and should always be thrown away.

Before a person injects the drug, he should swab the skin with alcohol, and again after the injection. While this might not seem important to stop the spread of HIV, it is important in keeping the person's skin healthy and intact. If the person is helped to remain as healthy as possible, and is informed of ways to ensure that HIV is not spread, he will pose less risk to society.

One of the greatest errors that can be made is failing to respect people who suffer from addiction. Easy to judge as lazy, difficult, and menacing, these men and women are more correctly victims of a dreaded disease. They are unable to stop without help; they have no choice. The drugs that are injected are some of the most potent and addictive of substances, and the ability to stop taking them is simply not there. It is not a valid response to the HIV epidemic to look at treatment success in terms of sobriety. In all other aspects of medical treatment, there is an effort made to enable the person to survive with the best chance of a cure. This means that the person who is not sober still should receive treatment, even though the outcome is not optimal.

Targeting Interventions

When a person is addicted to drugs and alcohol, he usually experiences problems that bring him into contact with health care workers, employee assistance program (EAP) personnel, and law enforcement officials. These workers and their agencies are in a perfect position to catch many of the people who are in trouble with substances.

The first concern is recognizing the addict. Many might think this is easy to do, but it is difficult. One of the most important things to remember is that using these substances is illegal, and the addict must therefore hide his use. In order to secure drugs, a person must be able to move in society without being noticed. Many of the people who use drugs do not fit the descriptions of those whom most people would think of as addicts or IDUs.

Case Study 7.9

"I started using [morphine] when I was a nurse. No one knew what I was up to, they all thought that I was trustworthy. I was not into getting high with people at work, so they never really knew that I was sick. I would wait until a patient was in the ward who was on morphine. There were always a couple. We were supposed to toss old drugs down the drain in the presence of another person, but things were always so busy that I just would say that I tossed it. It was no big deal because this was really the standard practice. I mean everyone did this, I mean toss the drugs out without a witness. It was so easy to get the stuff, and when I shot up I was okay. I mean that I was not out of control, I was calm and able to do my job. It was if I could not get any morphine that I would have problems, the shakes and the sweats, cramps and all that stuff.

"I was in the EAP worker's office twice about drug use. It came to their attention after I was caught by a coworker. I lost my job and started to cop on the streets. It was really something. After I got caught things were bad, not better. I started running with a man who was also into injection drugs. I tested positive after he died of hepatitis."

Susan, 35, registered nurse

Case Study 7.10

"I was never into drugs, so I never thought that I was at risk for something like HIV. I was really into my body and working out. When I was sick for the first time, I was not sure what the problem was. I started to lose some weight, and then I was waking up in my bed and I was soaked with sweat. I went to my doctor and they did a routine blood test and they saw that I had a T-cell count of 89. They tested me for HIV and I came back positive. I know that I got the disease from other guys at the gym who I used steroids with years ago. I never thought of this as a problem. That is, I never thought that this was a risk factor."

Jack, 33, sales representative

People who had an addiction, be it to steroids or drugs such as cocaine or heroin, all need to be thought of as people at great risk for HIV transmission. Identifying the person who is using drugs is often difficult, but there are some symptoms that can be recognized.

Identifying the IV Drug User

There are clues to identifying the drug user, and identification is the start of treatment or eduction, both of which are viable strategies for reducing the spread of HIV.

A person who is using intravenous drugs often has mood swings that are more severe than those seen in "normal" people. These swings are a direct result of the drugs. A person might go into the bathroom looking like a train wreck and emerge acting as though he is on top of the world. It is a misapprehension that the addict is always a person who is sitting in a doorway comatose from drugs. More often than most people realize, the drug user has a job and is able to function competently at work.

A person who uses drugs often has problems with his family life. He might complain about not being understood, and he will claim that he does not understand why people are upset with him.

Drugs are expensive, but a person will not do without them even if he cannot afford them. The addict will more likely allow his phone to be shut off than go without drugs.

IDUs are not likely to socialize outside of work with people who are not into using drugs. They are careful to avoid any behaviors or social activities that might show them in a different light and thus expose them as something other than a coworker.

There is often an alcohol problem as well, with alcohol being used as a way to level off the person after he gets high. The person might come into the workplace hung over at the start of the day, only to become better after he has gotten high. Simply put, the mood and the affect of the person might be extreme.

A person who uses IV drugs often will have sores where he has been injecting the drugs. He is not likely to allow them to be seen, and will even compensate by wearing long-sleeved shirts all the time.

The bottom line is that the only ways to truly ascertain if a person is using drugs is to elicit an honest answer (though this is unlikely), catch him in the act, or detect drug metabolites in urine screens. The signs that point to a substance abuse problem are: frequently missing work with undocumented excuses, erratic mood swings, financial difficulties, difficulties in personal relationships, and run-ins with law enforcement. While none of these indicates definitively that there is a substance abuse problem, it should not be ruled out.

The next issue then becomes what to do with the person who

is thought to be involved in substance abuse. The answer varies and should be investigated on a case-by-case basis. Calling a local, certified substance abuse treatment center is one way to start the process. Treating a person for substance abuse is a long and difficult process that requires a person to be engaged in ongoing treatment. Such treatment is of course beyond the scope of this book and should be addressed by a health care professional.

Like identifying the person who uses other drugs, identifying the person who uses steroids can be done, but it requires the ability to open the mind and see the symptoms for what they are. The user's family and social systems are often in denial about the situation and do not see the signs that in retrospect seem to be so clear.

Case Study 7.11

"My son had all the signs of a person who uses steroids. He started to gain body mass at a rate that was unusual. He would have mood swings, his hair started to thin, and he developed acne. At the time, we thought that he was just a big kid going through puberty. The signs of steroid use are so similar to growing up that by the time we figured out what was going on, we were too late. Scott killed himself with a shotgun. I am not sure if he shared needles, but the drugs that he took were as destructive as any of the illicit drugs that kids take."

MARY, 54, *mother*

This case study illustrates how the mind seeks to protect a person from a painful reality, a phenomenon referred to as *denial*. This is often the most difficult aspect to overcome in both the addicted person and his family.

A person who uses steroids is often thought of as "healthy" because he seems to be working out all the time and apparently watches his diet. The behaviors that are a part of the steroid user's world often mislead other people into thinking that he is not involved in behaviors that are dangerous; thus, there is little help available to him and less education to help prevent HIV transmission.

People who are involved in steroid use often have the following symptoms:

- Rapid muscle mass growth
- Rapid weight gain
- Thinning hair
- Increased and severe acne
- Mood swings
- Rage outbursts
- Obsession with body size

While these are common signs of steroid use, not all people
who exhibit these symptoms use steroids. It simply means that
they share the same behaviors as those who do.

Women and AIDS

In 1985, women made up 7% of all cases of AIDS in the United
States; ten years later, they made up 18%. In 1994, the number of
new AIDS cases in women accounted for 24% of all cases ever
reported in the population with AIDS.

The most frequent mode of transmission of HIV in women is
from the use of contaminated needles associated with injection
drug use, which accounts for 38% of all cases of HIV infection in
women. Following this risk behavior, heterosexual activity with
an infected partner is responsible for 38%. The remaining 21% of
HIV-positive women were infected through transfusions of HIV-
infected tissue products, or infection from unknown reasons, reported as "unknown risk."

AIDS in women is not egalitarian—it affects minorities more
than whites. While black and Hispanic women make up less than
21% of all women in the United States, they do represent 77% of
women with AIDS.

Finally, and most troubling, are the messages that promote
the idea that AIDS is not a major killer. These messages try to make
the incidence of AIDS appear smaller when compared to other

diseases such as cancer and heart disease; while this is true, it makes little impact when one realizes that AIDS is now the number one killer for black and Hispanic women, and the fourth leading killer of white women in the age group of 24–44 years. As HIV becomes more prevalent in the United States, it becomes important to look at the way that HIV affects women physically, emotionally, and financially.

HIV Infection in Women

In female populations, the most frequent AIDS-defining conditions are Candida esophagitis and Pneumocystis carinii pneumonia (PCP). The most commonly observed initial HIV-related symptoms are related to yeast infections: oral, esophageal, and vaginal.

Women also suffer from gender-specific pathologies. Many of these diseases were not recognized at the start of the AIDS epidemic because, first, the focus was not on women, and second, women of childbearing age have been excluded from most clinical trials since 1974, when then president Richard Nixon and the Food and Drug Administration (FDA) imposed restrictions that were meant to protect unborn children from possible side effects that were then unknown. The lack of female subjects in clinical trials has translated into a policy whereby women are not looked at today when health care issues are considered, as there are few data to support or refute their needs.

In 1992, the CDC began to look at specific female pathologies associated with HIV infection. Not surprising to women, of course, was the fact that there were diseases that were specific to their bodies.

Pelvic Inflammatory Disease

Pelvic inflammatory disease (PID) is a general, acute inflammation of a woman's pelvic cavity. It is not considered an HIV-defining illness, and it should be understood that PID also infects many women who do not have HIV, but severe cases are seen in women who have HIV. PID is caused from sexually transmitted diseases (STDs), commonly from a chlamydia infection.

Chlamydia is a microorganism that causes a variety of diseases, such as infections of the mucous membrane of the eyelids and the STD lymphogranuloma venereum, which is the most common STD in the United States.

Pelvic inflammatory disease can result in infertility and an increased risk of tubal pregnancy. Men are the primary carriers, but painful urination and discharge from the penis often prompts medical treatment, and often the disease has no symptoms that a woman would be aware of until the infection is well under way.

In women who have HIV, PID often seems to be more severe, causing a variety of infections, erratic menstruation, and severe cramps. While PID is not an indicator of HIV infection, women who have severe PID should be encouraged to take an HIV test.

In the following case study, Sarah, a 28-year-old bartender, tells how her severe PID led her doctor to investigate the possibility of HIV infection:

Case Study 7.12

I met Sarah in a hospice that works exclusively with people who are dying of AIDS-related diseases. Sarah was very thin, weighing under 90 pounds, and I could not see how tall she was, as she was lying in bed under a pile of blankets, which she told me helped her to stay warm.

"I had been out of a serious relationship for about three years, but I was sexually active with eight different men. I had no reason to think that I was at risk for HIV infection, because I lived in Buffalo, and I did not think that this was something that a woman would have to really think about living upstate, who was not a prostitute or druggie.

"I had started to really get some severe cramps and thought that it might be because I had gone off the pill ... the pill makes you less crampy," she told me as if she were letting me in on a secret.

"After the second month with these cramps, I went to Planned Parenthood to get back on the pill. When I saw the doctor, she told me that I had severe pelvic inflammatory disease. She told me that I should be tested for a bunch of sexually transmitted diseases. I felt so embarrassed. I always thought that the people who got STDs were sleazy, and here I was being told that I most likely had one. The doctor also suggested an HIV test. I remember thinking that this was not going to be positive, that just because I had a venereal disease did not mean that I was going to have AIDS," she said, and looked away from me.

"I came back to the clinic 13 days later, and they told me that I had tested positive. I was so stunned. I mean, I never thought that this was even a possibility; really, I thought that when all was said and done that I would have to take some medication and clean up my act. But here I am."

Invasive Cervical Cancer

HIV-infected women have a high risk of getting severe, invasive cervical cancer that is thought to be caused by the human papilloma virus (HPV), which is the cause of genital warts, and is a common STD that occurs in as many as 25% of women aged 25–35.

Women infected with HPV will often have squamous dysplasia, a precancerous condition. Many times this disease has no symptoms and is known to disappear. At the other extreme, it may develop into cervical cancer.

It is thought that the lower-functioning immune system, impaired by HIV, allows HPV to take a more aggressive hold on the body and thus be able to cause a more aggressive cancer. Invasive cervical cancer is much more virulent than the classic form of cervical cancer and, left untreated, will spread even more quickly and eventually cause death.

Yeast Infections

Vaginal yeast infections are fairly common in women because the moist, dark, warm environment of the vagina is conducive to the growth of yeast cultures. The infection that is associated with HIV is the same fungus that causes typical yeast infection. Candida infections become more virulent in women who suffer from

HIV infections because the immune system becomes so weak that it can no longer fight off funguses. Again, it should be noted that a yeast infection is not a sign or symptom of HIV infection.

While the physiological differences between men and women may account for some difference in treatment, policy, and life expectancy, there are many other factors besides the biological ones that change the treatment afforded to women.

Until recently, women have not been recognized in the AIDS epidemic. For example, early studies in women were limited to blocking maternal–infant HIV transmission. However, women now make up 13% of those with AIDS, and as this statistic continues to rise, there has been no unified attempt to remedy the primary focus of clinical research on men. There are few efforts to increase scientific understanding of how HIV affects women.

Understanding How Women Are Infected with HIV

As more and more women in society are infected with HIV, the importance of knowing how the virus is transmitted in women becomes increasingly evident.

During intercourse, there is a chance that there might be small cuts or tears in the vagina that would facilitate transmission of HIV from the man's semen to the woman. Even with no sores, however, it is still possible that a woman might be infected with HIV.

The exact mechanism that facilitates this infection is not known. The epithelial cells on the surface of the female genital tract lack a CD4 receptor. This suggests that HIV might not necessarily need CD4 receptors, but may prefer them. It is clear that CD4 cells are critical at the point of HIV infection, but it could be that the virus is able to use other mechanisms to ensure infection.

The Status of Women in Society

To understand the impact that AIDS has had on women, it is important to examine how an AIDS diagnosis excluded women during the first decade of the epidemic. An AIDS diagnosis is not based on a positive HIV antibody test, but rather on the presence of certain diseases in conjunction with a positive HIV test. Gender-specific diseases contracted by women with AIDS were not considered part of the AIDS diagnosis until 1992; therefore, women who had HIV and cervical cancer, for example, were not included in the statistics of women having AIDS. The reasons for this omission are complicated, but worth examining.

Gender Bias in American Medicine

Women have long been plagued by a double standard that permits sexual freedom to men but denies it to women. Because of this double standard, women's sexuality has been ignored or hidden by a society that prefers to promote the idea that "good women" are chaste and virtuous. For example, England's Royal Highness, Princess Diana, had to be a virgin in order to marry the Prince of Wales, while his own sexual history was never an issue.

Consider the role of women in prostitution, still an illegal act in all but one of the United States. In other words, when a man approaches a woman and sex is negotiated for a sum of money, both parties are breaking the law. However, both parties are not prosecuted equally. Moreover, the victimization of women through prostitution is rarely portrayed realistically. For example, the movies "Pretty Woman" and "Risky Business" portrayed prostitution in a completely unrealistic manner. While the film industry is not responsible for setting societal norms, it does often reflect them.

Given their unequal treatment and second-class status in the United States, women are simply overlooked when it comes to having the political and social clout to enact governmental change. They are severely underrepresented in all areas of government, with the result that policy platforms exclude women's issues, such as health care. In AIDS research, the focus has been on the male population afflicted with the disease. Therefore, research dollars have not been dedicated to exploring AIDS and women. So, their plight and connection to AIDS remains very much a troubling mystery.

Although AIDS research has increased enormously, it will take time to collect sufficient information on diseases contracted by women with AIDS. This means that there is currently no viable way to ascertain what type of risk AIDS poses to women.

Admitting that AIDS is an issue for women is the starting point. Many politicians and fringe groups believe that only gay men, promiscuous women, and drug users contract AIDS and HIV. This misinformation must be addressed and corrected. There are thousands of women with AIDS who were unaware they were at risk for contracting HIV. Consider the following case history of Doris, who is 46, HIV-positive, and afflicted with lymphoma:

Case Study 7.13

"I got HIV from a blood transfusion that I received after I had a hysterectomy. Ironically, now they say that I might not have needed the surgery. I became sick in 1988, but no one knew what was wrong with me. No one said it might be AIDS. For over a year, I was looked at by a lot of people before a medical student looked at me and asked if I had been tested for HIV. I was tested and it came back positive. It never dawned on me that I might have AIDS. I had received my transfusion after they started to screen blood for HIV. All in all, I feel railroaded into dying. I might not have needed the surgery that caused the need for me to get the transfusion, which gave me AIDS. It all has to do with how women are treated in our society and in medicine.

"If I had it all to do over, I would have been a lot more interested in women's affairs, like NOW and that stuff. I won't get the chance to watch my children grow up and see my grand-children. But I'll tell them that they can avoid all this. I tell my daughter and my son to get active in women's issues. I tell them that I am not dying because I have AIDS, but because I'm a woman. It's the same things for gays. They might die of AIDS, but they are dying because people don't care about them. The irony of this is really hard. I used to think that gays got AIDS because they were so promiscuous. It was that thinking that kept them in their gutter. And it's the same thinking that's going to secure me a grave. If I had looked at this as a disease, not a curse, I would've read more about it. I would have talked more about it. I would have fought for treatments.

"You know, there are people that think that AIDS was made by the government. It's silly, really. But it was certainly made worse by our irresponsible government. I watch the television now and I see the politicians. I listen to some of them, like that one Helms from the South. They should be ashamed, as should every sad little mind that votes to keep them in office. They do more to spread AIDS than gays and all the others that have been identified at risk. I used to play bridge. Things change."

The lack of treatment for HIV-infected women has caused many in the medical establishment to propose the creation of a certified medical specialty in women's health analogous to pediatrics or geriatrics. The specialty would have its own course of training in medical school similar to those for other specialties. Such a program would act to correct medicine's reliance on the male model as the medical norm for human beings. In addition, such a specialty would fuse the normal medical care for women, now split between the obstetrician/gynecologist and the general practitioner, with a single doctor responsible for reproductive, cardiovascular, and mental health.

The AIDS epidemic has emphasized the serious consequences of assuming that diseases develop in the same way in both sexes. More than ten years into the epidemic, the Centers for Disease Control and Prevention has finally added criteria for AIDS as it affects women. These uniquely female diagnoses, which were not caught, often caused a delay in medical treatment, and thus shortened women's life expectancy as compared with men's.

Furthermore, as they were not included as eligible for AIDS diagnosis, women were unable to qualify for public assistance, causing them additional economic hardship. This, however, is not the only issue that women must contend with. HIV-infected women often confront racism, sexism, classism, and lack of empowerment—a combination that can lead to isolation. In cases of divorce or single parenthood, women are often the custodial parent, and this further adds to the formula in the United States that keeps women poor and isolated, a deadly combination for those with AIDS or HIV.

Case Study 7.14

"I have worked with people who have AIDS for about three years. When I first started to work with this population, I did not really see a big difference between men and women. What I mean is that I did not see any more difference caused by AIDS than I had seen as a woman working in a male profession. Actually, I thought of myself as a liberated woman who has done pretty well for herself. Well, it really hit me how much men are not the parent when my daughter was born. I had just returned to work at the hospital, and a friend asked me if I wanted to grab some dinner one night that week after our shift.

"I was working in a clinic at the time, and it was pretty nice to have set hours. Rob, my husband, and I graduated from medical school together and had waited until we were both done with our residencies before we started our family. We had both talked about not raising a child in a world where we practiced any real bias stuff. Well, anyway, I had just started to work again and I was really excited about being back at work, I was actually glad to get some adult interactions in my life again.

"We had a woman come in and take care of Megan while we were at work. I was only working three days a week, and on these days Rob would come home before me, so that the baby-sitter could get home. So there was never an issue of me 'having to get home.'

"Well, I told my friend that I would have to see if Rob would mind baby-sitting. I mean REALLY, baby-sit! It's his child too. What do I mean, baby-sit? I mean Rob is great, it was me. I could not believe that I correlate baby-sitting and fatherhood."

JANE, 38, *family medicine practitioner*

Case Study 7.15

Scarlet, a 44-year-old homemaker with six children, is HIV-positive, as are three of her children. She was infected by her boyfriend, Peter, who is the father of the three youngest children. Eight months ago, Peter died of AIDS-related pneumonia at the age of 48.

"I cannot believe that this is happening to me and my babies. I wake up every morning and just look up at the ceiling thinking that this is the worst damn thing that could of happened. And I'll tell you I think that I am right too.

"I am starting to feel worse, and I know that it is this HIV. The doctors tell me my cells are down, and this means that I am getting sick, and this really gets me down. It's hard to get up and do the things that I have to do. I still have children that need things like shoes, and lunches for school, and clean clothes. I feel bad because soon I am not going to be able to do all that much. Soon I am going to have to have them go and stay with my sister because I cannot do it all any more. I have not told them this yet, and I know that it is what's going' to kill me.

"I mean I did not plan this. I didn't know that Peter would have this stuff. Man, it takes everything from you. But I just don't know how I am supposed to live when my family is all split up ... it's all going away, and I feel no peace. People have said that they think that it gets easier, but I don't think so. I think that it only gets harder to make it through this stuff, not knowing what is going to happen. It sure isn't easy."

Policy Setting for Women in the Age of AIDS

For all the struggles that women have to go through in the United States to be included in disease control and clinical research, it is a shame that when policymakers get their shot at helping the plight of women, they focus on women only as caretakers of children. Across the United States, there is a great deal of legislation that looks to help women with the problems associated with AIDS. Many of these bills are directed at women who are victims of sexual crimes, or they address issues involving children. The problem with policies that look to these groups of women is that there are limited resources, and laws that deal with the issues of rape and fetal testing either hurt women or do very little to their overall quality of life. The following situations dealing with screening tests objectively illustrate this phenomenon.

Since the first test for HIV was available, there has been discussion of who should be tested and the circumstances under which such a test be administered. After 15 years of battling the epidemic, there continues to be discussion of mandatory testing, especially that of newborn infants.

The debate that exists is not whether testing is called for, but rather whether or not the need for testing supersedes an individual's right to not take a test. If such a need is shown to exist, the issue that needs to be discerned from the myriad issues that surround testing people against their will, or at best without their consent, is how to develop an ethical standard that weighs equally the rights of the individual against society's need to know.

Newborn screening tests are routinely performed on infants for many diseases, specifically, inborn metabolic disorders, e.g., PKU and maple urine disease, among others. These tests are performed with the understanding that there are treatments available to those who are affected by the disease and that the tests will accurately diagnose the presence of pathology.

What is not often understood by many is that newborn infants do not produce antibodies, and therefore the screening exams, when performed, are not accurate measures of the infant's antibody status. Infants are dependent upon the antibodies they receive from their mother's body and milk, respectively, from gestation to 6–8 months postpartum. The tests performed on the infant will in fact reflect only the mother's antibody status. Statistically, 75% of those children born with their mother's HIV antibody will shed it by the time they are 18 months old, so in essence the child never was infected with HIV, making the test highly inaccurate.

These policies must, yet often do not, address the availability of treatments that can be administered to the child to prevent the onset of disease. Historically, screening exams have not included diseases for which there were no therapies. For example, Huntington's chorea, an inborn genetic disorder that affects 50% of all children born to an infected parent, is not screened for even though there are tests that can accurately diagnose who will have the disease. This disease, as well as many other known diseases that can be transmitted to children genetically, are not screened for simply because there is no available treatment. The point is that the policy governing screening tests supports the tenet that without treatment, the knowledge that these tests would bring is worthless. While it is easy to make black and white distinctions comparing diseases, such as PKU with Huntington's, the lines become more blurred when looking at HIV infections in newborns because there are no treatments available to the infected child. However, could there be less invasive methods available to detect the presence of the disease without jeopardizing the right to privacy from the woman's perspective?

Clearly, screening tests do not accurately detect the virus in newborns; thus, the rational for the screening test, that it can enable physicians to treat the child prophylactically, is flawed. Such plans advocate the administration of prophylactic treatment to all infants who test positive for HIV antibodies. The implications are clear: 75% of "HIV-positive" infants would receive unneeded services. The inference from this policy is that there is no other effective way of providing prophylactic treatment, yet this is not the case.

Clinical data support the view that PCP is unlikely to occur in infants under 1 year of age if their CD4 lymphocyte counts are above 200. Even so, conventional wisdom suggests that a CD4 count of 1500 is a reasonable level for initiation of PCP prophylactics to infants less than 1 year old.

One justification offered for the concept of administering PCP prophylactic treatment to all children deemed "at risk" by virtue of a positive newborn screening test is that it would be acceptable in cases in which a child would not otherwise be receiving medical attention adequate to monitor lymphocyte counts. By virtue of receiving the prophylactic therapy, the child would then be engaged in a health care system.

However, the government's action of looking after the health of the infant is clearly duplicitous of the parents' role as custodian. Society clearly accepts it as being the parents' role to protect children, as is demonstrated in the case of tuberculosis. TB is clearly more of a threat to the public's health in regard to casual transmission, yet we allow parents to decide whether their children are to be tested for the disease. In this example, society clearly respects the parents' rights and obligations to the infant by not taking actions to otherwise change or subjugate parental power.

Another argument that advocates a policy of "unblinding" the screening of HIV in newborns is that it would prevent postpartum infection of the newborn via HIV-infected breast milk. The incidence of HIV infection from mother to child is unknown in the United States. In other countries, it should be noted, mothers often nurse babies during and after teething (thus providing access to the child's bloodstream) and are more dependent on breast milk for nutrition. The result is an 18% rate of HIV transmission attributed to nursing. However, if this is the case, the testing should be conducted not on the infant, but on the mother. Therefore, it becomes necessary to challenge the constitutionality of the policy. It must be remembered that women are a protected class in the eyes of the federal government, which affords protection to "at risk" groups from pejorative and damaging behaviors. This requirement would challenge the constitutionality of the measure on the grounds that it puts an undue burden on women compared to men, and would require a higher standard for implementation of such policy.

Courts across the United States have made it very clear that men and women share equality under the law guaranteed by the Fourteenth Amendment of the United States Constitution. In several cases, the courts have addressed the issue of gender neutrality, consistently deciding that men and women are equal in regard to the law and its application. The law states that statutes that treat men and women differently violate equal protection unless the differentiation is substantially related to the achievement of an important governmental objective. Furthermore, the test should have a substantial relationship between the need to discriminate and the provisions of a policy to achieve that objective.

If the effect of these types of policies is to restrict the freedoms afforded to women, certainly the need should be extraordinary. The need in this case is statistically negligible, as it will prevent transmission in only a fraction of pediatric AIDS cases. If, then, the measure is the risk of infection posed to others, common sense and epidemiological data suggest that men should be tested, as they are the greatest amplifier for HIV in the United States, and therefore pose the greatest risk to the population. Furthermore, if restrictions of freedoms are to be imposed for the sake of the child, then it makes more sense to test women for HIV infection while they are pregnant, thus offering the child real protection and the best chances for being born without HIV. Doctors looking to reduce the rate of infection of HIV between mother and fetus administered zidovudine (AZT) as a prophylactic treatment, achieving a reduction in the rates of infection from 25.5% to 8.3%. Certainly, if the ethical catalyst for this policy is to look after the best interests of the child, then the ethical solution is to test pregnant women. However, the Fourth Amendment clearly states that people have a right to privacy despite the resultant issues as to whether or not a woman's body is private.

The Fourth Amendment to the Constitution clearly affords a level of privacy to all citizens. The "right to privacy" entails (1) the right to be left alone; (2) the right to exercise autonomy or control over significant personal matters; and (3) the right to limit access to the self. Clearly, both by design and by interpretation of case law, the Fourth Amendment is meant to protect citizens against "all invasions on the part of the government and its employees of the sanctity of man's home and the privacy of life." This includes one's body.

Summary

Homosexuality is the orientation of approximately 10% of society's members, whereby their primary intimate relationships are with people of the same gender. Until 1975, homosexuality was officially classified as a disease in the *Diagnostic and Statistical Manual of Mental Disorders*, published by the American Psychiatric Association, but is now known to be a normal and healthy orientation.

In the early 1980s, there was an explosion of AIDS cases that disproportionally affected the gay male population. Later, many would say that homosexuals introduced AIDS into the United States, though this was not the case. The stigma that AIDS brought to homosexuals was tremendous and further fueled the bias against this group.

Working with the gay client requires that a helping person be cognizant of the plight that gays and lesbians face in the workplace, government, and health care.

The incidence of HIV in the IDU population is a large source of HIV infection and is undoubtedly a major problem. Addiction is a medical disease that if left untreated usually ends in death. In the course of the disease, the afflicted person will often place himself in situations that can lead to further harm from a multitude of diseases, such as tetanus and hepatitis.

HIV is also an issue for women. While the effects of HIV on women are still unknown, recent efforts to look at women and their health are yielding more information on the way HIV infects a woman's body overall. The results of more surveillance of women and HIV only point out, sadly, that women who have unprotected sex with men put themselves at great risk for infection.

8

AIDS Education

To date, there is still no indication of a cure for AIDS. The only recourse is to educate people and hope thereby to prevent them from becoming infected. Most people agree with this mandate; however, controversy has arisen over educational methods. Doubts arise about whether it is better to promote safe sex versus abstinence; the appropriate age at which children should be educated about sex, AIDS, and HIV; and who the appropriate spokespersons are to deliver these educational programs.

These questions are met with conflict and judgmental attitudes. Many believe certain aspects of AIDS education to be inappropriate—particularly a frank discussion of homosexuality, sexual acts, and the promotion of condoms as a method to prevent infection.

A common mistake made by those attempting to deliver HIV prevention information is the failure to assess the educational needs of the audience. Before any program can be designed and implemented, it is important to examine what is known thus far about AIDS and HIV, the groups at risk, and the overall effects of the disease on different segments of society.

The medical community has substantiated that there is a disease called acquired immunodeficiency syndrome (AIDS) that kills 90% of the people who develop it. It is thought to be caused by a virus called the human immunodeficiency virus (HIV), which is known to destroy the immune system. Presenting these facts is not in itself controversial. It is perfectly acceptable to present this

information to every person with the cognitive ability to understand the concepts of disease and death. This information is therefore appropriate for school-age children. It is not necessary, however, for children to start learning about AIDS in kindergarten.

It is imperative to remember that part of the beauty of childhood is freedom from the worry all people encounter as they age
and their roles in society become more complex. The question of
usefulness also must be addressed. It is not useful to know about a
disease without understanding how to avoid it. Likewise, very
young children who are not at risk might not need to know how to
avoid disease transmission. However, older children do, and
those who are at risk need to know how to avoid becoming HIV-
infected.

AIDS is a disease that can be prevented. This should be the
mantra of all educators. As lawmakers and leaders begin to hear
this message, they will become more willing to allow the AIDS
educator access to the people who need to know about prevention, that is, everyone who has the physical capacity to engage in
behaviors that can transmit HIV.

Fear of sexuality often prevents AIDS education. Many leaders
in the field of AIDS education have their roots in groups that are
predominantly gay. Groups such as ACT UP were so powerful in
both education and policy making that many people believe an
AIDS educator is also a gay rights advocate. This is not the case. It
is important to give credit where credit is due, and if it were not for
the courageous efforts of many gay men and lesbians in our
society involved in ACT UP (and similar groups), the AIDS epidemic might be worse than it is today. Notwithstanding the contributions of these groups, many people remain homophobic, and
while ACT UP and others educate people about AIDS to promote
change and equality, this objective should be secondary to that of
preventing the actual disease.

Professionalism and AIDS Education

The greatest obstacle that homophobia would place in the
way of AIDS education is not that it would bar gay men and

lesbians from teaching children about HIV and AIDS. Rather, it is the assumption that anyone working in AIDS education must necessarily be homosexual. The approach taken must therefore be professional, to protect both the AIDS message and the messenger.

The first thing people see during an AIDS education presentation is the presenter. If the presenter looks "different," his appearance detracts from the message and is deemed unacceptable. If the presenter is dressed in jeans, a tee shirt, and freedom rings, there's a problem. A dentist wears a lab smock. The auto mechanic wears coveralls. Likewise, the educator who is discussing a health matter, not a political one, should dress as other health care educators dress. People educating others about AIDS need to know that the message, not the messenger, is the focal point of the HIV and AIDS program.

The tone of the presenter is the second most noticeable aspect of the presentation. Although humor can act as an icebreaker between the presenter and the audience, and can help make people less uncomfortable with realities that go hand in hand with AIDS and HIV infection, humor can also make AIDS and its victims seem less important. In short, there is nothing humorous about AIDS, and hearing about AIDS should perhaps make people a little uncomfortable. The presenter's tone should simply be open, understanding, and filled with authority.

Another aspect of tone is vernacular. Many would-be AIDS educators use words that are not appropriate, such as "cock" and "asshole." These terms may be the norm for certain groups, but they are not socially acceptable. One educator has said that such word choices seem to be more powerful and acceptable during presentations on college campuses. The speaker may think that this is the case, in a given situation, and it may very well be, but professionalism dictates that educators use words that are acceptable and pedagogically correct. The use of street language to describe activities of gay men and other devalued populations may be viewed as acceptable precisely because of the disrespect with which such people are viewed. There is a tendency to let the audience develop and dictate the limits of educational seminars concerning AIDS education and safe sex. This is not the preferred dynamic; rather, the educator should take the lead, while remaining aware of the audience throughout the process. The presenter, by resisting the temptation to be "cool" and instead maintaining a professional attitude by using appropriate terminology and adhering to social norms, helps allay the idea that those concerned about AIDS must be gay, or gay sympathizers. Presenters who adhere to social norms gain access to people and get their message across, which is the aim of AIDS education.

The foregoing ideas about a professional presentation apply in every situation. The educator must nevertheless vary his strategy and convey his message appropriately to the group he is addressing.

Presenting AIDS to Children Ages 9–12

Children are difficult to address about the issues of AIDS. They also comprise one of the most important groups to be targeted. Children between the ages of 9 and 12 are beginning another social chapter of their lives: entering junior high school.

In junior high school, the norms of behavior change. It is now acceptable to admit to liking members of the opposite sex. Peer groups become more coed. This time also marks the start of physical changes for many youngsters as they enter puberty.

It is not uncommon for children to know very little about sex and yet be reluctant to admit their ignorance. Thus, the presenter might be confronted with a group of people completely ignorant about adult sexual roles. It makes little sense to talk about AIDS and how to avoid contracting it if knowledge of actual intercourse is nonexistent or blatantly incorrect. This requires sex education, which can be unsettling for both children and parents.

Ideally, parents explain to their children, in a loving and nonthreatening environment, what sex is and how it can be a wonderful part of an adult's life. However, such ideal learning is not every child's experience. The gap between what a child knows about sex and what is real is the first thing a presenter must explore.

It is not the educator's responsibility to explain to this audience what sex is. Therefore, the presenter first needs to get in contact with the school leaders to find out if there is a sex education class, and if so what is being taught in the class. Parents should also be notified that a presentation is going to be held and informed of what is going to be presented to the audience. Doing so serves two purposes: It demonstrates, first, that there is nothing wrong with talking about AIDS to children and, second, that the AIDS presenter respects the rights of parents to be involved in all aspects of their children's health and education.

Presentations should be scheduled well in advance to allow ample time for parents to tell their children about sexual relationships. A letter should be sent to the parents recommending that they talk about sex with their children so the children will be able to understand the material being presented. In addition, this notice should indicate that the presentation encourages their children to remain abstinent from sexual intercourse; parents want to hear that their children are not being encouraged to engage in sex. While reputable educational groups have never encouraged children or young teens to have sex, the constant and powerful propaganda from the political right has led many parents to believe that such encouragement occurs during an AIDS education presentation. Pat Robertson, for example, has said that "what Planned Parenthood is doing is absolutely contrary to everything Christian. It is teaching kids to fornicate."

The presenter should also make himself available to parents with questions about the presentation materials or any concerns they might have concerning AIDS.

The Presentation

The presenter should be aware that many times the group of students will be uncomfortable with AIDS and its sexual implications. It is the presenter's job to address the issue first. Of course, it can be embarrassing to talk about sex and sexual behaviors. Just admitting that it is embarrassing often clears the air. The presenter should then define AIDS by explaining the acronym AIDS: Acquired Immunodeficiency Syndrome. Each of these words should be defined:

- *Acquired* means that it is not something we are born with, or that is a part of our being, but rather is the result of exposure to an agent.
- *Immuno-* refers to *immunity*, which is the body's way of protecting us from infection and disease.
- *Deficiency* means that there is something lacking, so that the immune system cannot do its job.
- *Syndrome* is the name given to a disease, like AIDS, that has many symptoms and ill effects, not just a few.

The next step is to explain what causes AIDS. First define HIV and how it attacks the body. Then explain that the cells in charge of fighting diseases (the white cells) are the same cells that HIV attacks. As the virus continues to attack these cells, other diseases attack the body.

This is often a very complicated concept for younger people to grasp. Using an analogy from everyday life may help them conceptualize how this disease works. For example, blood cells can be compared to the members of a football team. The defensive linemen (white cells) keep the other team's offensive line away from their end zone. The quarterback does not fight the other team because he has another role. Imagine that all the defensive linemen are injured, and because of their injuries they begin to weaken and lose the game.

Telling children the truth about the outcome of AIDS is often difficult. But the truth is that the majority of people with AIDS die from the disease, and children have a right to know what the consequences of certain behaviors could be.

The next aspect of educating children about AIDS is explaining the ways in which it is spread or transmitted: through sexual contact, receiving contaminated blood products, and sharing needles.

Explaining Sexual Contact

The presenter must be aware that a great deal of sensitivity is needed to convey this point to young adults and children. The fact that AIDS is not caused by sex should be stated repeatedly to the group. Many times, for an adequate presentation, it will not have been assumed that the parents have provided the necessary background, and the presentation will therefore include the basic facts about sex.

Defining sex is often the most difficult aspect of a presentation to adolescents. Children at this age are aware of their anatomy; they know that boys have penises and girls have vaginas. It can simply be explained that each of these organ systems produces cells that when mixed together can produce another being. The way these two types of cells are introduced to each other is through intercourse, in which a man places his penis into the woman's vagina.

The presenter should explain that sex is ideally a part of adult relationships. People have sex because they enjoy the intimacy it can bring to partners who love each other. This type of intimacy is a very adult feeling, and not appropriate for children. Explain that there are many adult feelings that children and young adults do not yet understand. Likewise, children have feelings that adults don't. It is important to say that it's okay to think about sex, and to ask questions, but it's not okay to have sex at a young age. It is very important to state that having sex at a young age can cause a girl to become pregnant and can subsequently cause her to be at risk for HIV.

It should be noted that having sex at a young age not only puts a youngster at risk for contracting HIV or a host of other diseases, but also creates tremendous pressure and emotional strain.

The presenter should encourage children to talk about their feelings and to ask questions about sex with a responsible adult such as the school nurse, an older sibling, or ideally a parent.

This presentation should introduce children to the danger that HIV poses to everyone as well as how to be kind and accepting of those who have HIV. A noteworthy example of the consequences of prejudice is the experience of the Ray family of Arcadia, Florida. The family was afflicted with the genetic disorder of hemophilia, which is characterized by the inability to stop bleeding once it begins. The treatment for this ailment is to administer blood transfusions. In 1987, it became known that the three Ray boys had contracted HIV from transfusions. The community's response to their plight was horrific—they refused to let the children attend school, burned their home, and chased the family out of town. This was brutal behavior, and the pain inflicted upon the Rays was immeasurable. The hatred that these children were subjected to was fueled by misinformation, fear, and ignorance.

It is crucial for children to understand that people with AIDS, aside from their illness, are like anyone else. It must be stressed that befriending a person with HIV is a good thing. AIDS is not a punishment, nor does it affect only gays and drug users. It is a virus that can affect us all. Stressing to children the commonality of all people leads to an understanding that most of us want the same things in life.

Accepting others is another aspect of presenting HIV to young adolescents. There are gay people in this world, as there are people of different races and religions. Simply because a Catholic befriends a Jew doesn't mean one of the two has to switch religions to have a true friendship. Likewise, a heterosexual can befriend a gay person without turning gay. The belief that talking about homosexuality is in fact "recruiting" is absurd. People do not choose their sexual identity. Teaching children that accepting and valuing others makes the world a better place is hardly recruiting.

Adults are responsible for protecting children, including gay children, who suffer from a higher incidence of suicide and substance abuse, facts forgotten by those in education and government. If educators are successful in promoting a healthy sense of self in all children, the results will be rewarding enough. Children and adolescents with a healthy sense of self have a lower incidence of drug abuse, promiscuity, and failure to complete school. This does not mean that the presenter advocates particularly for gays and lesbians, but rather insists on a policy for all people to have the right to be treated with kindness and equality. This is an important message in a society in which there are far too many negative messages concerning the value of homosexuals in modern society.

Education Summary for Children Ages 9–12

Before any educational program is implemented, it is important to first review the curriculum of the host organization:

1. Explain to the group what AIDS is and what causes it.
2. Explain that sexual intercourse can lead to AIDS if one of the partners has HIV.
3. Explain that sex is not appropriate for people of this age group.
4. Encourage children to talk about AIDS, sex, and drugs with their parents.
5. Explain that all people have the right to be cared for and valued.
6. Allow time for questions.

It is also important to contact all parents and allow them time to talk with their children about the impending presentation.

AIDS and HIV Presentation for a High School Group

Young adults need to be educated about sex and sexually transmitted diseases. Since research indicates that the majority of young people will engage in sexual intercourse during their high school tenure, it is important that schools open their doors to the professional HIV and AIDS educator. Many people are doubtless unaware that the number of high school students with AIDS is low, but the number of people in their 20s with the disease is much greater. This means that many of these people were probably infected with HIV during their teenage years. It is a responsible and moral action for adults and educators to give teens the information they need to make informed decisions and to take proper precautions.

When presenting HIV prevention information to teens, it is important to contact parents to make them aware that a program on AIDS will be delivered. Remember that while many of these "children" stand over six feet tall, they are still loved and cherished babies in the eyes of their parents. If the educator initiates the presentation process with respect for the family and educational system, there is a greater chance of gaining access to teens.

It is also important to examine the school's stance on sexual education. Who runs this curriculum? What is taught, exactly? Working within an already established school curriculum will streamline the task at hand. Developing a working relationship with school administrators will allow continued access for presentation of AIDS education programs.

Sexuality is undoubtedly one of our most powerful drives. Wisdom and prudence do not often prevail when someone is sexually aroused. This lack of judgment is not just common to teens. Adults in all age groups experience mistakes in judgment where sex is involved. The goal of educating young people is to help them recognize their limits. All teenagers are experiencing sexuality and the desires that go along with it. The educator who conveys an understanding of these new feelings is a powerful ally.

Most young people today are under many stresses. The added stress brought by an intimate relationship can often be overwhelming. By and large, it is recommended that children of high school age abstain from sexual activity. However, it is not a perfect world, and many teens do engage in sexual activity. Educators, parents, and health care workers therefore need to be frank about sexual behaviors and practices.

Review with the teen group all sexual practices and inform them of the risks each holds. Explain that simply because an activity is called low risk does not mean that it poses no risk. If a person engages in an activity that has risk, then there is a chance he may contract HIV and AIDS. These factors or behaviors are not always commonly understood; three people may hear the same words but take three different messages from them. This miscommunication occurs when a speaker does not explain the words he uses.

Sexual Behaviors

In presenting information on sex, make it clear that although other people continue to have sex and take risks, it does not mean theirs is the example to follow. That is to say, the educator is not encouraging sex between teens, but rather stating facts. The relative risk associated with various sexual behaviors, as outlined below, should be conveyed to young adults.

- *High-risk behaviors*: Vaginal and anal intercourse.
- *Lower-risk behaviors*: Oral sex, "French kissing." There is no real evidence that deep kissing can spread AIDS, but it is theoretically possible.
- *No-Risk behaviors*: Masturbation, touching, and hugging.
- *Safe Sex*: Any behavior that does not involve the exchange of body fluids. Two messages teens need to hear are (1) that it's okay *not* to have sex, but (2) if they choose to have sex, they should approach a doctor, nurse, or counselor about safe sex practices.

Condoms

Prevention through condom use has been highly debated. Whether or not it is appropriate to make condoms available to sexually active teens and young adults lies at the center of the controversy. Does making condoms available to teens encourage sexual promiscuity and activity? The answer is no.

Children raised with love and respect grow to understand that sex is a special part of being an adult. Some will wait, others won't. Sex at a young age might very well be a big mistake, but it should not cost a life. Because children can lose their lives as a result of sexual activity, we need to have condoms available to sexually active teens.

Educators must explain that the use of a condom does not guarantee that a sex act may be performed with no risk of HIV transmission. There are questions about the effectiveness of condoms, even when they are properly used. Latex is imperfect as a barrier, because it tends to have microscopic holes that can apparently be larger than the HIV virus.

In addition, condoms are not strong enough to withstand certain sex acts and have been known to tear. There are also questions about what brands of condoms are effective in stopping HIV transmission. Natural condoms, those made from animal membranes such as sheepskin, are not effective in stopping HIV. Latex condoms are more effective than natural condoms, but are often used incorrectly. For a latex condom to provide the most protection, it must be worn correctly and applied with a water-based lubricant.

College Presentations

Presenting information about AIDS and HIV to college students is similar to presenting to high school students in that the talk should be frank and open. Presenters often give people tips on how to spice up their sex lives in ways that do not put them at risk for transmitting HIV. This is unprofessional and unnecessary. Outlining how the disease is spread is more than enough.

Likewise, a banana (or other such object) should not be used as a representation of the penis to illustrate how to use a condom. Education about AIDS and HIV is a serious matter. Humor masks the fact that AIDS is a deadly disease; it is one of the greatest killers of young people to date.

Presenters also should talk to college-age adults about the hazards of drinking in terms of the effect of losing inhibitions about sex. What a person does after having a few drinks is often very different from what that person would do in the sober light of day. Drinking has long been a part of college life, and to ignore it is to ignore part of the AIDS dynamic. When people are drunk, they engage in casual sex more frequently. People socialize in bars for a reason. Alcohol lowers people's inhibitions and allows them to act more freely. In combination with AIDS, this disinhibition can be deadly.

Presenters also should talk to college students about being tested for the HIV virus. Testing is free in most states, and can offer a great sense of peace from knowing whether or not HIV is present. Unfortunately, many will get results confirming they have been exposed to the virus. This news is not entirely negative. The person who has tested positive has the advantage of being fore-warned to seek out medical advice before a crisis arises. A presen-ter should be fully aware of the testing procedure and how the tests are read and interpreted. A listing of area testing facilities is also a key component in presenting HIV and AIDS information.

Young people should be told that if they are participating in a sexual relationship, they should remain monogamous and get to know their partner. A new term currently in vogue is *serial monog-amy*, meaning that a person has one exclusive partner after an-other. The act of going from one relationship to another without protection is no different from picking up people in a bar. Those having sex only in the confines of a loving relationship are there-fore also at risk. An educator must stress testing before engaging in sex. The test should take place 6 months after the last sexual encounter.

Summary of Presenting HIV and AIDS to College Groups

- Define AIDS.
- Introduce HIV and how it infects the body.
- Explain how HIV is transmitted.
- Discuss safe sex.
- Testing.
- Questions.

Educating Groups Thought to Be at Risk

The term *risk groups* is a frightening one that gives those who are not members of such a group a false sense of security. It also separates people already on the fringe of society. Nonetheless, there are groups that do need special attention from health care workers, doctors, and educators, as well as more kindness, support, and validation from society. The rewards will be fewer deaths from AIDS and emotionally healthier people in subsequent generations in the risk groups.

Gay Teens: The Hidden Minority

Gay teens have a greater propensity for suicide and drug abuse than the rest of the population. They are not often visible or outspoken. The challenge for the AIDS educator is how to reach these children.

To effectively reach the gay teen, the educator must understand that young gay people have very little incentive to identify themselves in society as gay people. There is little protection from the cruelty often directed at homosexuals in our society. The offhand use in our society of such terms as "fag," "homo," "queer," and "fairy" confirms to gay youths that they are not liked or appreciated. The gay teen is isolated from many social situations centered around heterosexual paradigms. For the young adult without sexual feelings toward the opposite sex, this is another message validating the view that they are different. The adolescent years are filled with anxiety. Growing up as a gay teen only magnifies this stress.

Often, the individual's process of acknowledging and accepting his sexual identity only invites more complications. It is very difficult for any teen to assimilate into his or her overall identity the new sexual feelings that adolescence brings. This difficulty creates a stressful time not just for the teens themselves, but for parents, educators, and other family members as well.

In our society, it is likely that children have gotten the message that being gay is bad. Gays are depicted as effeminate and silly on television and in most films. There is an absence of lesbian images except in pornography, where lesbian sexual acts are used to "turn on" adult males. In short, children have been exposed only to the horrific prejudice that society holds toward gays and lesbians. In school, where being different is fervently avoided, it makes little sense for the teen to identify himself as gay.

True identification means sharing self-identity with family members. This may prove to be an experience of anger and denial, so the teen chooses to hide his identity from those who love and trust him. The inability to acknowledge oneself without fear of ostracization from a peer group and the fear of telling the family cause enormous stress, and the results can be disastrous. So the question is how to reach gay teens who have so much invested in keeping their sexuality a secret.

The educator must realize that many gay teens won't seek help. To acknowledge themselves as gay means exposing themselves to ridicule and separation from friends and family. While this might not happen, it is a valid perception of risk. Gay teens aren't going to identify themselves, so adults must be made responsible for reaching this group.

Often, the first health care professional sought out by adults needing information and guidance on what they have come to realize of their child's different sexuality is their child's pediatrician. It is important that pediatricians become familiar with issues facing gay teens in our society and be willing to talk to parents about having a child who is not heterosexual. Doctors must realize that a gay teen needs special attention. This does not mean that the gay teen is emotionally unhealthy. What is crucial to understand is that gay adolescents are at greater risk of harming themselves physically or through drug abuse. Parents must acknowledge that gay children do exist. A gay child may not be their child, but it could be a nephew, a niece, or a friend's child.

Teachers need to be aware that some of their students may be gay, and take the responsibility of ensuring that such students are afforded an equal opportunity to perform at optimal ability. The following case study illustrates the high school experiences of Brian, now aged 18, a freshman at a state university who is involved in the university's gay and lesbian association.

 Case Study 8.1

"I was 13 when I really started to know that I was gay. I knew before then that I was different. But I wasn't sure why. I had crushes on guys before, but they weren't sexual. My family knew I was different, and so did all the kids in the neighborhood. Kids were mean to me. I think they knew that I was different. But, like me, they didn't have a name for it. I was mean then, too. At one moment you were good friends with someone, and the next you were on top of them beating the shit out of them. It was really odd. But I think that's the way it is for all kids. I was pretty lucky, really. I had a cool brother and sister, and my parents were pretty nice.

"When I was about 13 I started the 'change.' I remember I was getting more and more sexual. I was getting pubic hair and a lot of erections. A few of my friends were starting to get really into sex and would read dirty magazines. We would all look at them and talk sort of dirty. I was more interested in the guys than the women in the photos. I never let on and would talk about fucking girls and the whole ball of wax. I remember I was starting to masturbate, and I was thinking about men, not girls. This really disturbed me, but I still was unaware that there was such as thing as gay men.

"Somewhere around this time, my sister told me that a guy in town was gay or a fag. I'm not sure, but she used some term like that. I was confused and asked her what she meant. She told me that he liked guys … liked to have sex with them. I was shocked, but I kind of knew too. It was during this point that I really started to have major bouts of depression. I was only 14 but I was so depressed. I thought a lot about killing myself and ways to do it. But I would always feel kind of guilty about those thoughts, so I held back. I can honestly say that I really wished I was dead then.

"I started high school and things became really tough. Kids started to pick on me and call me names. I think they knew. Things at this point really became brutal. I was constantly picked on and ridiculed. I was punched every day by a group of guys. I would come home with bruises on my arm. Teachers would see this, and I think that they convinced themselves that it was just a good ol' time. I'm not sure how they came to this conclusion. I'm sure I looked scared.

"The entire situation just kept getting worse and worse, so I stopped going to school. I would skip school every day, and then get in trouble. I tried to tell my parents about what was happening, and they thought I was just making excuses. It was really screwed up. I was forced to go to a place where I was beat on and ridiculed for eight hours a day. I was always afraid. For four years of my life, I was afraid—I mean really afraid. I knew at this point that I was gay, but no one else really knew. The bullies kind of knew that I was different. I started to skip school again. This was not a delinquent behavior. It was survival. I mean, kids would scream out that Brian is a fag. Not a single person would tell them to stop. They would tell me, however, to get thicker skin! It was really screwed up. Blame the victim.

"In eleventh grade, I met a guy in school who was also gay. We started to hang out a lot, and then we became sexually involved. It was one bright light in my four years of hell. But there were problems. We would fight, in the mean way that lovers fight, and there was no one that I could talk to about this. My parents came to me and started to question why we, Kevin and I, were always together. I would make up lies, saying we were just good friends. Things started to sour between us, or maybe more accurately, around us. There were still people calling us fags, and the like, but having someone to go through this with made it seem easier. By the time we were seniors, things were getting better, mostly because I could see that high school was ending. Man, it was like the Emancipation Proclamation. I was free from these goons.

"In April of my senior year, Kevin shot himself in the head. I was in Boston at a college interview, and when I returned home with my dad, my mother was sitting in the kitchen. I knew when I came into the room that something was up. She told me point blank, and I think in a way she was relieved. I think they knew what was going on, and I think that she was glad that he was away from me. I don't mean to say that she was glad that he died, but she was glad that he was away from me.

"It really killed me. I cried and cried. I'll never forget what it was like to go back to school. People were really nice to me for the first time. I think that they were only nice to me because they were feeling guilty because they were a part of his death. Today I really hold them, meaning the entire community, teachers and students, responsible. I mean he was a great kid and the other kids destroyed him, and the teachers let it happen. It was sick. I'll never forget what it was like, knowing that the person I loved most at that time was in such pain that they had to kill themselves. It was so obvious, the crap we went through every day. No one did anything to stop it. It was murder. After a few months I started to get really depressed. I felt that there would never be anyone that understood me, or my loss. Back then I didn't know what was causing these sad feelings; it just seemed that the entire situation was so dark.

"My parents came to me and asked me if I was gay. I think that they knew before this, but they never had the courage to ask. I was so tired of it all I told them that I was. At first they were quiet. They had to digest it, I think. Then slowly they started to become really angry about it. It was more than I could take. I mean I was only 17 and had been ridiculed and picked on for four long years. I was trying to get into college and deal with the loss of my best friend and lover. I was so tired at 17, it felt more like I was 90. My parents and I started to fight a lot. It wasn't over being gay, but little things like not making beds or keeping my room messy. It was all a front to justify their anger and hatred that I was gay. They were really concerned for me as well. I think that they were not only angry about me not being a perfect son who gets married and has kids, but they were worried that I would kill myself like Kevin did, or that I would get AIDS. There is a lot to be scared about.

"We started family counseling before I came here. It was really great. The counselor started out by saying that being gay was not the problem. For the first time in my life, I heard that I was not the sick one, the problem. It was very freeing for me, and I think for my parents as well. No one had told them that it was okay that their kid was gay. When I look back on things now, I think that I was a great kid with great coping skills, but I needed someone to tell me this. At times I think of Kevin, and I think that he would have really liked college and being around other gays and people who accept us. It's like Utopia, but that's not the case. I still think that what happened in high school was a crime. I still have so much anger toward some of the teachers and administrators. They still tell people that they're not responsible for Kevin's death, that he made a choice. I suppose he did, but it wasn't a real choice. They beat him till the only choice he had was to kill himself.

"If you use this in your book, I want people to know that a guy killed himself because all he got out of his life was crap and hate from people. To be a gay teen means that there's no net out there for you. It sucks and it's still like that today. No net, no one out there saying that kids are killing themselves because the message from all around says they are bad and sick."

When giving a presentation to groups of young adults, excluding information germane to gays and lesbians is sidestepping the fact that these are the teens most likely to be afraid to openly identify themselves. As this case study illustrates, gay teens have already learned that the very part of their nature that puts them "at risk" is not to be revealed. At times, the gay teen believes that his very survival depends on keeping his homosexuality a secret.

Discuss the notion of choice in sexuality. The idea that there is a choice is a damaging message to present to a young person struggling with his sexuality. It not only makes the gay youth aware that he is different but also implies that this difference is wrong and that he can change himself and has responsibility for his sexuality. That kind of responsibility is not assigned to the heterosexual young person. Every educator must understand that the gay teen is no more responsible for his sexuality than he is for his eye color.

Gay youth are not at risk for HIV infection because they are gay. A lack of self-worth allows gay teens to engage in activities that put them at risk for AIDS as well as a host of other diseases. Gay teens are starving for appreciation and acceptance. It is easy for them to fall into a pattern in which pleasing a partner becomes more important than self-preservation.

Like other teenagers, gay teens need to socialize. In some large metropolitan cities, youth centers are provided for this population, but they are uncommon elsewhere. Without a safe place to explore and define their sexuality, gay teens gravitate toward places that are not safe for young people. Bars and clubs have historically been the places where gays and lesbians socialize. Bars serve alcohol, so they are not safe places for young people to socialize. However, they remain one of the few places where gay teens can go to meet people like themselves. Mixing alcohol with feelings of inferiority and alienation is disastrous. The supervision and authority present in many heterosexual social situations are often missing in the gay teen's social structure.

The final component of the gay teen dynamic is the issue of sexual practices. It is often ignored by parents, teachers, doctors, and counselors. The heterosexual teen is constantly bombarded with messages to wait until marriage before engaging in sexual intercourse. These teens are well versed in the roles men and women adopt during intercourse. The gay teen has none of these benefits, lacking both the ceremony of marriage and defined sexual roles. Gay teens need to be guided about what is acceptable sexual behavior in their relationships.

Peer interaction is an important part of constructing a sexual identity. Talking about the "hot" girl or the "cute" guy is a wonderful aspect of being in a social world. Gay teens, though, don't have access to this interchange, and so develop feelings of isolation and loneliness.

Information should be made available about gay and lesbian groups that are accessible and provide privacy and guidance. School health officials should talk about healthy sexual practices that are relevant to both homosexual and heterosexual groups. All schools should establish policies that address hate-motivated crimes, thereby sending the message the bigotry has no place in education.

Administrators should devise programs that help teachers deal with their feelings about gay and lesbian youth. Teachers should know how to recognize conflict and prejudice. They should know how to teach children that prejudice is unacceptable. Children should be required to attend a seminar in which they can explore violent feelings and find a method to vent these feelings that is not at the expense of other students.

What Parents Need to Know

Adolescents believe life is endless and they are invincible, untouchable, and free from harm. But research indicates that many people with AIDS today were infected when they were teenagers. How then do parents reach adolescents about the seriousness of AIDS? How can parents make teenagers understand that a night's fun could potentially end their lives?

A young person is more at risk today than ten years ago. AIDS is the number one killer of young adults in over 20 cities in the United States. This number has risen every year since public health officials began to record the number of AIDS deaths.

What the Kids Need to Hear

Explanations about sex and reproduction are often badly delivered. The following scenario depicts the confusion or misinformation to which an adolescent may be exposed:

Case Study 8.2

"When I as about 11, we were going to see a sex education flick in school. They sent home a letter telling my parents that the film was going to be shown about reproduction, and that our parent should talk to us about sex. I was really in the dark about sex. God I don't think I had given it much thought before then, where babies came from. Well, I knew that they came from a girl's stomach, but how they got in there I wasn't at all sure. Well, my mother told me that a girl has eggs and a guy has sperm. The guy takes this sperm and puts it on a girl's egg and a baby is born. The next day I shared this with the guys in school. My interpretation was: A guy puts sperm on an egg. Where the sperm came from I had no idea. I thought that the egg came from a hen or something. Then the guy puts the egg up the girl's vagina. This was what I thought sex was from my mother's discussion. Needless to say, I learned a lot about the differences between my version and the real McCoy. The movie cleared it up, but they never talked about how the sperm got from the testes to the vagina. However, I got the point of fertilization. I tell you, though, thank God for the kids in the back of the bus. They knew the real deal ... I think their parents were hippies."

Often, a parent's inability to successfully explain sex and reproduction furthers the message that sex is wrong and should remain hidden. To prevent this from happening, parents must address both sex and sexuality. It is important to raise children with healthy and open minds about sexuality so that they will be able to make prudent and wise decisions about sexual behaviors.

Sorting Out the Differences between Sex and Sexuality

Sex is a motivating drive in all people, a fact that is often overlooked by parents relative to their adolescent children. Parents may encourage their children to abstain from sex—and this message may be followed. However, there still remain relevant issues that must be discussed with adolescents.

It is negligence not to inform youngsters that sexuality is a complicated and emotional component of adult relationships that involves a commitment on the part of both individuals. Without this information, youngsters can minimize their accountability and responsibility for their actions. Rarely are the powerful and emotional aspects of sexual relations shown to our young people. The baseless image of sexuality pumped through the mass media often serves as the only sex education adolescents receive. Given this situation, how can young people be expected to avoid behaviors that are dangerous and laden with intense emotions, and often result in disastrous consequences?

Parents must realize that talking about sex and sexuality typically does not encourage sexual activity.

What Young Adults Need to Know about Sexuality and Sex

The very first concept young adults need to know is that it is okay to acknowledge sexuality. Parents must discuss and process with their children not only information about sex, but also thoughts and fantasies that arise at many times and situations. Explaining the subtleties of sexuality will encourage responsibility in young people. Most parents fear their children will become involved in sexual behaviors that may lead to pregnancy, diseases, and promiscuity. These are all realistic fears, but keeping young people in ignorance will not prevent these tragedies from occurring.

Masturbation is often the first sexual experience for young adults. While there is little risk for disease transmission in this act, it is an act that is often connected with shame and pathology. Adolescents must be informed otherwise.

There are many books that have been sensitively written for adolescents about early sexuality and desire. Often, just the knowledge that sexuality is natural and not perverted may ensure a healthy start on the road toward adulthood. Allowing the young adult to experience his sexuality without shame is certainly a very good preventative measure for some of the problems associated with poor self-image and sexual shame.

Pornography is a common introduction to sexuality. Finding such material in the possession of an adolescent can provide a wonderful opportunity to skip the all too common lecture and instead talk to the child about sex and sexuality. Acknowledging that such materials promote sexual arousal should be part of the discussion. The danger of regarding people as sexual objects should also be discussed. This does not mean that adolescents should not look at attractive people with lust. Parents need to explain that it is often the hidden aspect of a person that makes them sexy, and the great fun and fulfillment of sex is sharing it with a person one knows, both physically and emotionally. This encourages young people to search for intimacy and trust in relationships that involve sex.

It is also important that parents stress to young people that any intimate act requires trust. Kissing is truly exciting when those involved truly know one another. By instilling in young people that trust is an important criterion for an intimate relationship, certain risks that young people face are reduced. Trust is an important component in the development of healthy relationships. Allowing a teenager to question without fear is a powerful foundation of trust. There is nothing wrong with questioning what sex is, how often people have it, and what role sex plays in the life of an adult. Explaining that sex is to be cherished is one way of conveying to young people that it is not to be freely given away.

When young people begin to date and socialize, sex becomes an issue. This does not mean that they are having intercourse. The emotions associated with an adolescent's first physical relationship are often difficult to process. Feeling isolated and alone with these feelings often encourages a sense of urgency and "togetherness" between the two young people. Dismissing feelings as "puppy love" doesn't help the young people involved. Their feelings are real and powerful, and often very pure. Parents need to acknowledge this and respect the developing relationship. Doing so demonstrates that the parents trust the young person's feelings as special.

In an environment of trust and respect, the lines of communication tend to remain open. A young person who talks to his parents about his relationships gives the parents an opportunity to provide feedback and support.

What Young People Need to Know about Birth Control

Parents have been debating for years the merits of providing young people with birth control. AIDS and HIV, however, have made the issue more pressing than ever. Regardless of a parent's stance on premarital sex and birth control, unprotected sex could result in AIDS. The majority of parents agree that while sex at a young age is a mistake, it is definitely not worth dying for. While parents might wish, plead, beg, and pray that their children abstain from sex until they are older, their doing so will not guarantee abstinence.

Parents who believe their child is sexually active need to discuss birth control. Making birth control available is not permission or encouragement, it is simply a responsible reaction.

A parent has to take the lead in exposing young people to birth control measures. It is also important to understand that birth control does not mean safe sex. Birth control is any device or method that prevents the conception of a child. A device or procedure that protects a person from HIV infection during sex constitutes "safe sex."

Condoms: What Parents Need to Share

Unfortunately, the mass media have conned the public into thinking that condoms are the passport to safe sex in today's age of AIDS. What is often not explained is that for condoms to be effective, certain steps must be followed, and even then, absolute effectiveness still is not guaranteed.

The first thing parents should know is that not all condoms are the same. A natural skin condom is not effective in reducing the risk of disease infection. These condoms have many pores that allow the HIV virus and other small particles to move freely through the membrane.

The latex condom is most effective and should contain a spermicide called monoxail-9. Condoms should not be old or stored in extreme heat or cold, and should be rolled over the penis, leaving a small amount free at the tip to collect the ejaculation. If a condom is rolled tightly across the tip of the penis, it could break. Water-based lubricants should be used with a condom because petroleum-based jellies will break the latex down and not prevent infection.

After the male ejaculates, he should remove his penis from his partner's vagina or anus while holding the condom at the base to prevent it from slipping off. Condoms used carefully are the most efective way to reduce the risk of HIV infection during intercourse.

Certain brands of condoms are more effective than others. A study conducted at the University of California at Los Angeles (UCLA) compared different brands and ranked them on the basis of a variety of criteria, including tests of water and air leakage, tensile strength (elasticity), and other factors. The results are presented in Table 8.1.

Condoms and Leakage of HIV Virus

The UCLA condom study also subjected 14 condom brands to additional tests to specifically determine if they would permit leakage of HIV.

Table 8.1. Ranking of Condom Brands in the UCLA Study

Rank	Average score	Brand name	Manufacturer
1	92.5	Mentor	Mentor Corp.
2	89.5	Ramses Sensitol	Schmid Labs
3	88.9	Ramses non-lubed	Schmid Labs
4	87.9	Gold Circle Coin	Circle Rubber
5	86.0	Gold Circle	Circle Rubber
6	86.0	Sheik Elite	Schmid Labs
7	78.0	Durex Nuform	Schmid Labs
8	76.8	Trojan-Enz	Carter-Wallace
9	74.9	Lifestyles Stimula	Ansell Americas
10	70.9	Pleaser	Circle Rubber

Tests were conducted on the eight brands of latex rubber condoms that scored highest in the study's initial ranking of 31 brands and the five latex brands that scored lowest.

One brand of natural lambskin condoms—Fourex Natural Skins—was also tested to determine whether that material allows passage of the HIV virus. Tests were conducted on 10 condoms of each brand using a machine that simulates the stresses of actual intercourse.

All eight of the highest ranking brands successfully prevented passage of the HIV virus. They included:

1. Mentor by Mentor Corp.
2. Ramses non-lubed by Schmid Labs
3. Ramses Sensitol by Schmid Labs
4. Gold Circle Coin by Circle Rubber
5. Gold Circle by Circle Rubber
6. Sheik Elite by Schmid Labs
7. Durex Nuform by Schmid Labs
8. Pleaser by Circle Rubber

The following four of the five lowest ranking brands in the original study leaked the HIV virus:

1. Lifestyles Conture by Ansell Americas
2. Trojan Naturalube by Carter-Wallace
3. Trojan Ribbed by Carter-Wallace
4. Contracept Plus

Summary

The safest method of preventing transmission of HIV is abstaining from sex. If this is not an option, then there are other protective methods that can be used to help prevent HIV transmission. It is very important to know a partner's history. To do so calls for frank and open discussions about prior relationships and behaviors. Young people who are going to have sex should seek out a professional person to whom they can talk about contraception methods, protection from sexually transmitted diseases, and possible consequences that may arise from a sexual relationship. Doctors and professionals at local family planning centers are well versed in dispensing such advice.

If you, the reader, are a parent, then it is probable that you are concerned and willing to take action to protect your child from HIV infection. Many parents, however, are not. There are many children who are not raised in a milieu in which they are valued individuals. These children are starved for love and attention. They often have no education or supervision. How, then, do parents protect their children from peers who may not have the same information? The reality is that as long as unprotected sex continues, everyone is at risk.

How can parents protect their children? One way is by motivating schools and other agencies that serve young adults to implement educational programs that reach all young adults.

Educational programs that inform students about HIV and the measures to prevent infection have been attacked by many groups as a way of encouraging sex in teenage populations. This is not the case. The principle that parents giving information about sex promotes responsible behavior can also be applied to this situation. Providing adolescents with information about HIV and how to avoid infection during sexual relations is not irresponsible.

Sound educational programs include information about sexually transmitted diseases, unwanted pregnancies, emotional effects of sexual activity, and risk-reduction methods.

Parents and educators should avoid programs that attempt to scare young people about sex. Fear is not a healthy preventive measure. Adolescents need to learn how to make healthy choices.

Another important aspect of sexual education often ignored by parents is homosexuality. Few programs address the issue of gay teens. Doctors rarely talk to parents about the possibility that their child might be homosexual. When a child identifies himself as not heterosexual, he is identifying himself as having different educational and emotional needs than most of his peers. A gay child is at more risk for many problems than are his heterosexual peers. To address these issues is not to encourage a sexual preference.

Parents of gay children face many difficulties that parents of heterosexual children do not have to confront. Often, parents of gay children feel responsible for their child's sexual identity. Parents of gay children also face certain losses: In many cases, their children will not get married or have children.

However, gay and lesbian people can have very fulfilling lives. The fact remains that there are many more similarities than there are differences between gay people and heterosexuals.

All parents must insist that AIDS and HIV education programs include information about homosexuality and disease prevention. Many people have both same- and opposite-sex relations in their lives. If parents do not support gay and lesbian sex education, then they are in fact denying real protection to all teens and sexually active people.

Parents of gay teens also face questions about their children's social lives. For example, what is appropriate for the gay teen in terms of dating? The very same limits placed on a heterosexual teen are appropriate for the gay teen. Although there aren't many resources for gay and lesbian teens in most communities, there are some. Telephoning gay and lesbian community centers is one way of locating information about gay and lesbian activities that are designed for teenagers.

Parents often need support and assistance in accepting that their son or daughter is homosexual. Many areas have groups for parents who need support during their child's coming-out process. Parents and Friends of Lesbians and Gays (PFLAG) is a nonprofit group that conducts meetings that address many of these issues in a safe and supportive environment, and its services are free.

Telephone numbers for AIDS information are provided in Appendix A. Appendix B lists publications in the areas of AIDS treatment, prevention, and research.

Glossary

Absolute CD4+ cell count (T4 count): The actual number of T helper cells (lymphocytes) in a cubic millimeter of blood. The CD4+ count is significantly lower in HIV+ persons.

Acanthamoebiasis: Infection with *Acanthamoeba castellani*, a free-living amoeba that ordinarily inhabits moist soil or water.

Accrual: The process of signing people up to participate in drug trials.

Acquired: A condition not inherited or congenital.

Acquired immunodeficiency syndrome (AIDS): A disease believed to be caused by a member of a virus from the retrovirus group called HIV (human immunodeficiency virus), of which there are a number of variants that also may cause AIDS.

Active immunity: Immunity produced by the body in response to stimulation by a disease-causing organism or other antibody.

Acupuncture: Therapy in which needles are inserted into the body at specific points called meridians. The precise disorder to be treated or the degree of anesthesia required determines the temperature of the needle used, the angle of insertion, and the speed of insertion and withdrawal.

Acute: Rapid in onset; severe, life-threatening. The opposite of persistent, chronic, or long-term.

Acyclovir (ACV) (trade name Zovirax): A prescription and antiviral drug used to treat herpes simplex. Some studies suggest that ACV given with AZT may increase the anti-HIV benefit of AZT.

Addiction: Physiological and psychological dependence on and craving for a chemical substance.

Adenocarcinoma: Technical name for a malignant tumor derived from a gland or glandular tissue, or a tumor composed of gland-derived cells that form glandlike structures. Examples include most cancers of the colon, breast, pancreas, and kidney, and many other organs.

Adenopathy: Enlargement of glands, especially the lymph nodes.

Adenovirus: A group of DNA-containing viruses.

Adjunct: Any substance that is taken in conjunction with, and used as a treatment secondary to, a main treatment.

Adjuvant: Any substance that enhances the immune-stimulated properties of an antigen or the pharmacological effect of a drug.

Aerosolized: A form of administration in which a drug, such as pentamidine, is turned into a fine spray or mist by a nebulizer, and inhaled.

Agent: Any substance or force capable of bringing about a biological, chemical, or physical change. An agent can also be a person acting on behalf of someone else.

AIDS clinical testing unit (ACTU): The sites at which the AIDS drug clinical trials of the National Institute of Allergic and Infectious Diseases are performed.

AIDS-related complex (ARC): A term, not officially defined or recognized by the CDC, that has been used to describe a variety of symptoms and signs found in some persons infected with HIV. These may include recurrent fevers, unexplained weight loss, swollen lymph nodes, and/or fungus infection of the throat and mouth. Also commonly described as *symptomatic HIV infection*.

Allergen: Any substance that causes an allergy.

Allergy: An immediate or delayed immune reaction caused by the presence of foreign antigens.

Allogeneic: Having cell types that are distinct and cause reactions in the immune system.

Alopecia: Transient hair loss resulting from use of certain therapies.

Alveolar: Pertaining to the alveolus (plural *alveoli*), the air cell that is the site of gas exchange in the lungs. Alveoli are approximately 0.25 mm in size, and there are approximately 1.5 million in each lung.

Amebiasis: Infection caused by a tiny animal parasite, *Entamoeba histolytica*, which lives in the human large intestine.

American Medical Association (AMA): The largest physician-oriented organization in United States medicine.

AmFAR: The American Foundation for AIDS Research, a private, nonprofit agency based in Los Angeles, California, that raises funds for AIDS research.

Amino acid: Any one of twenty or more organic acids, some of which are the building blocks for proteins and are necessary for metabolism and growth.

Analgesic: An agent that reduces pain without reducing consciousness.

Analog or analogue: A chemical compound with a structure similar to that of another but differing from it in respect to a certain component; it may have a similar or opposite action metabolically.

Anaphylactic shock: An often severe and sometimes fatal systemic reaction in a susceptible individual upon exposure to a specific antigen (such as wasp venom or penicillin) after previous sensitization that is characterized especially by respiratory symptoms, fainting, itching, urticaria, swelling of the throat or other mucous membranes, and a sudden decline in blood pressure.

Anemia: A condition in which there are not enough healthy red blood cells in the bloodstream or too little hemoglobin in the red blood cells.

Anorexia: Prolonged loss of appetite that leads to significant weight loss.

Antibacterial: A substance that stops or slows the growth of bacteria.

Antibiotic: A substance that kills or inhibits the growth of organisms and is used to combat disease and infection.

Antibody (Ab): A specialized molecule in the blood or secretory fluids that tags, destroys, or neutralizes a specific bacterium, virus, or other harmful toxin.

Anticoagulant: A substance that delays or counteracts blood clotting.

Antiemetic: A drug that prevents or stops nausea and vomiting.

Antifungal: A substance that kills or inhibits the growth of a fungus.

Antigen (Ag): A foreign protein that can cause an immune response by stimulating the production of antibodies in the body.

Anti-inflammatory: A substance that counteracts or suppresses inflammation. There are two types: steroidal agents, such as cortisone, and nonsteroidal agents, such as aspirin or colchicine.

Antiprotozoal: A substance that kills or inhibits the growth of protozoa.

Antiretroviral: A substance that stops or suppresses the activity of a retrovirus such as the HIV. AZT is an antiretroviral drug.

Antitoxin: An antibody that recognizes and inactivates a toxin produced by a certain bacterium, plant, or animal.

Antiviral: A type of substance or process that destroys a virus or suppresses its pathogenic action.

Asymptomatic infection: An infection, or phase of an infection, without symptoms.

Asymptomatic seropositive: Infected with HIV but showing no apparent symptoms.

Ataxia: Loss of muscle control leading to jerky or uncoordinated movements.

Atrophy: A wasting or decrease in size.

AZT: See *Zidovudine (ZUD)*.

Bactericidal: Capable of killing bacteria.

Bacteriostatic: Capable of inhibiting reproduction of bacteria.

Bacterium (plural bacteria): A microscopic organism composed of a single cell. There are many kinds of bacteria, many of which can cause disease when they infect someone.

Basal cell carcinoma: A common skin cancer.

Baseline: A known value with which later measurements can be compared (e.g., baseline temperature, baseline hemoglobin level).

Basophil: A type of white blood cell, also called a *granular leukocyte*, filled with granules of toxic chemicals, that can digest microorganisms.

B cell: One of the immune system cell types; B cells fight infection primarily by making antibodies.

Benign: Of mild type or character that does not threaten health or life, as in benign tumor.

Bioavailability: The rate and extent to which a substance is absorbed and circulated in the body.

Biological response modifier (BRM): A substance, either natural or synthesized, that boosts, directs, or restores normal immune defenses. BRMs include interferons, interleukins, thymus hormones, and monoclonal antibodies.

Biopsy: Removal and laboratory examination of tissue from the living body.

Biosynthesis: The building up of a chemical compound in the physiological processes of a living organism.

Blastogenesis: The process of producing newly matured lymphocytes (a type of white blood cell) in response to a challenge by infectious agents such as bacteria and viruses.

Blastomycosis: An infectious disease caused by a fungus, usually in the lungs. It can spread to the skin, bone, or other tissues.

Blood–brain barrier: A barrier between brain blood vessels and brain tissues that restricts what may pass from the blood into the brain. This barrier presents a problem in treating HIV infection because treatments must cross it to stop HIV infection in the brain.

B lymphocyte (B cell): One of the two major classes of lymphocytes. During infections, these cells are transformed into plasma cells that produce antibodies specific to the pathogen.

Body fluid: Term used for any of a number of fluids manufactured within the body. Usually refers to semen, blood, urine, or saliva.

Bone marrow: Soft tissue, located in the cavities of the bones, in which blood cells, including erythrocytes, leukocytes, and platelets, are formed.

Bone marrow cell pool: Those bone marrow cells responsible for the production of blood cells.

Bone marrow suppression: A condition that can be caused by certain drugs. It leads to a decrease in white blood cells, red blood cells, and platelets, a decrease that can in turn lead to bleeding or infections.

Bradykinesia: Difficulty in initiating, or a lack of, movement, often used interchangeably with *akinesia*; it is one of the four hallmarks of parkinsonism.

Bronchoscopy: Visualization of the trachea and lungs with flexible fiber optics. Often used as a diagnostic tool for PCP, which now can be diagnosed by a noninvasive procedure called *sputum induction*.

Cachexia: General ill health and malnutrition. A general weight loss and wasting occurring in the course of a chronic disease or emotional disturbance.

Cancer: A large group of diseases characterized by uncontrolled growth and spread of abnormal cells.

Candida: A yeastlike fungus that is commonly found in the normal flora of the mouth, skin, intestinal tract, and vagina, but can become clinically infectious in immunocompromised people.

Capsid: The protein covering of the nucleic acid core of a virus.

Carcinogen: Any carcinogenic (cancer-producing) agent or substance.

Carcinogenicity: The ability of a chemical or physical *agent* (drug, radioactivity, X rays) to facilitate the development of cancer, generally after a long latency period.

Carcinoma: A malignant tumor that may spread to other parts of the body.

Cascade: The continuation of a process through a series of steps. Each step initiates the next step until the final step is reached. The action may or may not become cumulative as each step progresses.

Case–control study: An epidemiological method in which persons with a disease condition are compared with a healthy population similar in age, sex, race, and other characteristics to determine the differences between them.

Catheter: A tubular medical device for semipermanent insertion into canals, vessels, passageways, or body cavities to permit injection or withdrawal of fluids or to keep a passage open.

cc: Abbreviation for *cubic centimeter*.

CD4 (T4): The protein embedded on the surface of helper T cells and other white blood cells to which HIV attaches itself. Also found to a lesser degree on the surface of monocytes/macrophages, Langerhans cells, astrocytes, keratinocytes, and glial cells.

CDC: Centers for Disease Control and Prevention, a federal health agency that is a branch of the Public Health Service.

Cell: The smallest independent unit of an organism. A cell is composed of *cytoplasm* and a *nucleus* and is surrounded by a *cell membrane* or wall.

Cell membrane: The wall around a cell that separates it from its environment.

Central nervous system (CNS): The brain and spinal cord with their nerves and end organs that control voluntary acts.

Cerebral: Of or relating to the brain.

Cerebrospinal fluid (CSF): A fluid that circulates around the brain and spinal cord.

Cervical dysplasia: Abnormal tissue development of the lower part of the uterus; may progress to cancer of the uterus.

Chemotherapy: The use of one or more chemical *agents* in the treatment of a disease.

Chlamydia: A bacterial infection that causes urethritis, conjunctivitis, and a variety of other symptoms. Chlamydia occurs as a venereal disease independently of AIDS, but can also appear as an *opportunistic infection*. Left untreated, it can lead to cancer.

Chromosome: A threadlike structure in the nucleus of a cell that contains genetic information encoded by *DNA*.

Chronic: Continuous or persistent; of long duration.

Clinical: Based on observation of the condition of patients and their symptoms, as opposed to blood work or other laboratory tests.

Clinical trial: A test to see how well a new drug works on people.

Coccidioides immitis: A species of fungus that can infect the lungs of people with AIDS, but can also spread to the skin, gastrointestinal tract, and central nervous system.

Coccidioidomycosis (California disease, desert fever, desert rheumatism, San Joaquin Valley fever, valley fever): A fungal disease caused by infection with *Coccidioides immitis*.

Cofactor: A substance, microorganism, or characteristic of individuals that may influence the progression of a disease or the likelihood of becoming ill.

Cognitive: Relating to awareness with perception, reasoning, and memory.

Cohort: A group of individuals sharing a statistical factor in a demographic study.

Colitis: Inflammation of the colon.

Colon: The part of the large intestine that extends from the cecum to the rectum—the last three to five feet of intestine; also called the *large intestine* or *large bowel*.

Colonoscope: A long flexible tube, containing fiber optics, used to perform colonoscopy.

Colonoscopy: Examination of the *colon* using a *colonoscope*.

Coma: A state of unconsciousness in which movement and mental processes are impaired. People in deep coma cannot be aroused by an external stimulus.

Complete blood count (CBC): A series of tests including cell counts, hematocrit, hemoglobin, and cell volume measurement.

Condyloma: A venereal wart caused by the papilloma virus. Condylomas exist as venereal infections independently of AIDS, but the *immunosuppression* of AIDS may cause them to proliferate.

Conjunctiva: A membrane that lines the inside of the eyelid and touches the white part of the eye; secretes a mucus that lubricates the eyeballs.

Contagious: Capable of transmitting infection by casual contact from one person to another.

Cornea: The outermost layer of the three tissues that make up the wall of the eyeball; the clear, transparent, curved portion that covers the colored part of the eye; enables light rays to enter the eyeball.

Cortex: The external part of an organ, such as the brain, kidney, or adrenal gland.

Cotton wool patches: White spots in the internal layer of the retina (the back lining of the eye). These spots indicate areas of blocked blood supply.

Cranial nerve: One of twelve pairs of nerves in the brain.

Cryptococcal meningitis: A fungal infection caused by *Cryptococcus neoformans* that affects the three membranes (meninges) surrounding the brain and spinal cord.

Cryptococcosis: An infectious disease seen in HIV-infected patients that is caused by the fungus *Cryptococcus neoformans*, which is acquired via the respiratory tract.

Cryptoccus neoformans: A fungal parasite that can infect the lungs of people with AIDS and may spread to the meninges (linings of the brain and spinal cord), lungs, kidneys, and skin.

CT: Abbreviation for computed tomography (CAT scan).

Culture: The growth of microorganisms or living tissue in the laboratory, in solutions that promote their growth.

Cutaneous: Pertaining to the skin.

Cytomegalovirus (CMV): A virus related to the herpes family. CMV infections may occur without any symptoms or may result in mild flulike symptoms of aching, fever, mild sore throat, weakness, or enlarged lymph nodes.

Cytoplasm: The watery material between the nucleus and the *membrane* of a *cell*.

Dehydration: The state produced by abnormal loss of body water, the deprivation or loss of water from the tissues. Dehydration may arise from an inability to drink either because of difficulty in swallowing or because the person is weak, drowsy, or comatose from any cause.

Delirium: A clouding of consciousness in which perception is disordered. The person is often restless, anxious, and inattentive. Hallucinations, both auditory and visual, occur and add to the person's distress.

Dementia: Chronic intellectual impairment (loss of mental capacity), of organic origin, that affects a person's ability to function in a social or occupational setting. AIDS-related dementia may be caused by HIV or other opportunistic infections such as *CMV*.

Dermatitis: Inflammation of the skin.

DNA (deoxyribonucleic acid): A complex protein in the nucleus of a cell that contains the cell's genetic code and is the carrier of genetic information. HIV can insert itself into a cell's DNA and use cellular mechanisms for replication.

Dysfunction: Poor functioning or abnormal functioning of a cell or organ of the body.

Effective drug: According to the FDA, a drug that is of benefit for a specific disease.

Efficacy: Strength, efficiency; the ability to achieve a desired effect.

EIA (enzyme immunoassay): A blood test to determine HIV infection. See *ELISA*.

Electroencephalogram (EEG): The record of the electrical activity of the brain obtained by means of the electroencephalograph.

Electrolyte: One of the electrically charged salts found in blood, tissue, fluids, and cells, including the salts of sodium, potassium, and chlorine.

Electron beam therapy: A type of radiation therapy.

ELISA (enzyme linked immunosorbent assay): A testing method to detect antibodies to HIV. It does not detect AIDS, but only indicates if viral infection has occurred. Also see *Western blot*.

Empirical treatment: Treatment undertaken when a precise diagnosis cannot be made, based on experience with similar cases.

Encephalitis: Inflammation of the brain, usually viral but sometimes bacterial in origin. Symptoms include headache, neck pain, fever, nausea, and vomiting. Nervous system problems may occur, such as laziness, paralysis, weakness, and coma.

Endemic: Associated with a particular locale or population group.

Endocrine glands: The organs in the body that are responsible for producing hormones.

Endogenous: Relating to or produced by the body.

Endorphinergic: Endorphinlike or endorphin-related. See *beta-endorphin* for a description of *endorphin* activity.

Endorphin: One of a group of hormones including beta-endorphin, metenkephalin, levenkephalin, and dynorphin.

Endoscopy: Viewing the inside of a body cavity with a device using flexible fiber optics.

Endothelial: Pertaining to the endothelium, the lining of the blood and lymphatic vessels, the heart, and other body cavities.

Endothelial cell: One of the cells that comprise the endothelium.

Endotoxin: A toxin present inside a bacteria cell.

Enteric: Of or relating to the intestines.

Enteric pathogen: A disease-causing organism that infects the gastrointestinal tract and sometimes spreads from there to other parts of the body.

Enteritis: Inflammation of the intestines.

Enzyme: A protein chemical that can accelerate a chemical reaction in the body.

Eosinophil: A type of white blood cell, called a *granulocyte*, that can digest microorganisms.

Epidemic: An outbreak of a disease among a population.

Epidemiology: The science concerned with the determination of the specific causes of distribution of a disease and of the interrelation between various factors determining a disease.

Epitope: A unique shape or marker carried on the surface of an antigen that triggers a corresponding antibody response.

Epstein-Barr virus (EBV): A herpes-like virus that causes one of the two kinds of mononucleosis (the other is caused by *CMV*). It infects the nose and throat and is contagious. EBV lies dormant in the lymph glands and has been associated with Burkitt's lymphoma, a cancer of the lymph tissue, and hairy leukoplakia.

Erythematous: Red or reddened.

Erythrocyte: A red blood cell, the primary function of which is to carry oxygen to cells.

Esophageal/gastric candidiasis: A fungal infection of the esophagus (gullet) and/or the stomach that often produces pain with swallowing and weight loss; an AIDS-defining opportunistic infection.

Esophagitis: Inflammation of the lower part of the esophagus, the tube that connects the throat and the stomach.

Etiology: The study or theory of factors that cause disease.

Exogenous: Developed or originating outside the body.

Exotoxin: A toxic substance made by bacteria that is released outside the bacterial cell.

Experimental drug: A drug that has not been approved for use as a treatment for a specific condition in a specific population.

False negative: An erroneous test result that indicates that no antibodies are present when in fact they are.

False positive: An erroneous test result that indicates that antibodies are present when in fact there are none.

Fatty acid: One of a group of lipids found in animal fats. Some fatty acids are essential for good nutrition.

Festination: A tendency to take shorter, quicker steps in walking. Like micrographia (handwriting becoming smaller in a sentence), it is a sign of Parkinson's disease.

Fibroblast: Any cell from which connective tissue is developed.

Floaters: A floating dark spot within the field of vision. Floaters can be caused by CMV retinitis, but also appear in some persons as a normal part of the aging process.

Food and Drug Administration (FDA): The agency of the federal government responsible for the regulation of drugs.

Fungus (plural *funguses* or *fungi*): A general term used to denote a class of microbes including mushrooms, yeast, and molds. Fungi cause infections such as thrush, cryptococcal meningitis, and *PCP*.

Ganglion: A mass of nervous tissue, composed principally of nerve-cell bodies, usually lying outside the central nervous system.

Gastroenteritis: Inflammation of the lining of the stomach and intestines.

Gastrointestinal: Relating to the stomach and intestines.

Gastrointestinal intolerance: Inability to take a drug because it causes problems in the digestive system, such as stomachaches or diarrhea.

Gene: A unit of DNA that carries the code for specific cell functions.

Genital: A sexual organ.

Genome: The DNA code that comprises the complete genetic composition of an organism.

Gland: An organ that produces specialized chemicals, such as hormones, that are released into the blood to act at distant sites.

Growth factor: A factor that is responsible for regulating cell proliferation (rapid and repeated reproduction), function, and differentiation. Different growth factors elicit different responses from different cell types, such as stimulating cell growth, enhancing cell survival, initiating cell migration, and stimulating the secretion of tissue-specific hormones.

Hairy leukoplakia: A whitish, slightly raised lesion that appears on the side of the cheeks, gums, or tongue; thought to be related to *Epstein-Barr virus infection* (an OI).

Half-life: The time required for half of a given amount of a drug to be eliminated from the body.

Helper–suppressor ratio: The ratio of helper T cells to suppressor cells.

Helper T cells (T4, CD4): One of a subset of T cells that carry the T4 marker and are essential for turning on antibody production, activating cytotoxic T cells, and initiating other immune responses.

Hematological neoplasm: A tumor of the blood-forming organs.

Hematotoxic: Poisonous to the blood or the blood-producing bone marrow.

Hemoglobin: The protein in red blood cells responsible for oxygen transport. Normal hemoglobin values are 12–15 g/100 ml for women and 14–16.5 g/100 ml for men. These values can vary.

Hepatitis: Inflammation of the liver caused by one of several agents; often accompanied by jaundice, enlarged liver, fever, fatigue, and nausea.

Herpes zoster: A condition characterized by painful blisters that generally dry and scab, leaving minor scarring. Also known as *shingles*, it is caused by reactivation of a previous infection from varicella-zoster, the virus that causes chicken pox.

HHS: Department of Health and Human Services, a branch of the federal government.

Hickman catheter: A flexible needle-shaped tube that can be surgically placed in a large blood vessel and held in place for a long period of time.

Histological: Pertaining to the science of tissues, including their cellular composition and organization. It usually refers to the examination of biopsies with a microscope.

Histoplasmosis: A fungal infection caused by inhalation or ingestion of spores of *Histoplasma capsulatum*. It causes acute pneumonia and inflammation of the meninges, heart, peritoneum, adrenals, and all other organs of the body. Symptoms usually include fever, shortness of breath, cough, weight loss, and physical exhaustion.

Hormone: An active chemical substance formed in one part of the body and carried in the blood to another part of the body.

Hypersensitivity: A condition in which the body reacts with an exaggerated immune response to drugs or other substances.

Hypo-: A prefix meaning lowered or reduced; below.

Idiopathic: Without known cause. For example, of the two major types of Parkinson's disease, the postencephalitic variety is associated with an attack of encephalitis, but the idiopathic variety has no apparent cause.

Idiotype: One of the unique and characteristic parts of an antibody's variable region, which can itself serve as an antigen.

IDU: Abbreviation for injection/intravenous drug user.

IgA: An immunoglobulin found in body fluids, such as tears and saliva, and in the respiratory and gastrointestinal tract, that protects the body's entrances from infection.

IgD: An immunoglobulin that is poorly understood, but is thought to participate in regulatory functions.

IgE: An immunoglobulin that participates in allergic reactions.

IgG: An immunoglobulin that circulates in the blood and enters tissues.

IgM: An immunoglobulin that primarily kills bacteria in the blood.

Immune complex: A cluster that is formed when antigens and antibodies bind together.

Immune system: The collective term for the complex functions of the body that recognize foreign agents or substances, neutralize them, and recall the response later when confronted with the same challenge.

Immunity: A natural or *acquired* resistance to a specific disease. Immunity may be partial or complete, long-lasting or temporary.

Immunization: Protection against disease by vaccination, usually with a weakened form of a pathogen that is unable to cause illness.

Immunodeficiency: A breakdown or inability of certain parts of the *immune system* to function, making a person susceptible to certain diseases that would not ordinarily develop.

Immunomodulation therapy: A therapy that attempts to reconstruct or enhance a damaged immune system. Examples of immunomodulation therapy for AIDS include DNCB, isoprinosine, and Imuthiol (DTC).

Immunosuppression: A state in which the function of the body's immune system has been reduced.

Incubation period: The time interval between the initial exposure to infection and appearance of the first symptom or sign of disease.

Infection: The state or condition in which the body (or part of it) is invaded by an infectious agent that multiplies and produces an injurious effect (active infection).

Intractable disease: A disease that is unresponsive to treatment.

Intravenous (IV): Within or into the veins. Intravenous drugs are injected directly into the veins.

Jaundice: Yellow pigmentation of the skin and whites of the eyes caused by liver disease (such as hepatitis) or excessive destruction of red blood cells.

Kaposi's sarcoma (KS): A cancer characterized by masses of small blood vessels that grow rapidly. Kaposi's sarcoma was initially thought to be a tumor of small blood vessels. Usually appears as pink to purple, painless spots on the skin, but may also occur internally in addition to or independent of the skin lesions. Originally seen in elderly men or in equatorial Africans in a slow-growing form. It can be accompanied by fever, enlarged lymph nodes, and gastrointestinal problems (an *OI*).

kg (kilogram): A measure of weight equal to 2.2046 pounds.

Killer cell: One of a class of immune system cells that function to kill cancer and virus-infected cells; also called *natural killer cell*.

Kupffer cells: A specialized macrophage in the liver.

LAK cell: A lymphocyte transformed in the laboratory into a *lymphokine-activated killer* cell, which attacks tumor cells.

Langerhans cell: A dendrite cell in the skin that picks up an antigen and transports it to the lymph nodes.

LAS (lymphadenopathy syndrome): A chronic enlargement of the *lymph nodes*, often associated with HIV infection.

Latency: The period when an organism is in the body and not producing any ill effects.

Legionnaires' disease: A disease caused by the *Legionella pneumophila* bacterium. It is characterized by high fever, gastrointestinal pain, headache, and pneumonia. There may also be involvement of the kidneys, liver, and nervous system.

Lentivirus: One of a subfamily of retroviruses that is cytopathic and causes chronic diseases.

Lesion: Any pathological or traumatic discontinuity of tissue, which may cause a loss of function (of the affected or surrounding tissue).

Leukocyte: Any white blood cell. Leukocytes play a major role in fighting disease. *Lymphocytes* are one subclass of leukocytes. The two types of white blood cells commonly associated with AIDS are *T cells* and *B cells*.

Leukopenia: A lower than normal level of *leukocytes* (white blood cells) in the blood.

Lipid: A substance extracted from animal or vegetable cells by "fat" solvents.

Lumbar puncture: A test in which cerebrospinal fluid (CSF) is withdrawn and analyzed (spinal tap). A small opening in the spinal column is made by a needle, to remove spinal fluid or to inject anesthesia or medicine; it need not be painful if enough local anesthetic is used.

Lymph: A transparent, slightly yellow fluid that carries lymphocytes. Lymph is derived from tissue fluids collected from all parts of the body and is returned to the blood via lymphatic vessels.

Lymph node: One of the small, bean-sized organs of the immune system, distributed widely throughout the body. Lymph fluid is filtered through the lymph nodes, in which all types of lymphocytes take up temporary residence.

Lymphocyte: A type of white blood cell, comprising between 20% and 50% of white blood cells in an adult. Lymphocytes are produced in the lymphoid tissues of the body. The B lymphocytes produce antibodies that are released into the bloodstream. The T lymphocytes, on the other hand, carry antibodies on their own surface and produce cellular immunity.

Lysis: Rupture and destruction of a cell.

Macrolide: One of a group of antibiotic drugs.

Macrophage: A type of phagocyte that acts to identify foreign material within the body, engulfing the material and then expressing on its own surface the specific chemical marker that can be recognized by other cells of the immune system.

Macula: The pigmented central area, or "yellow spot," of the retina devoid of blood vessels; it is the most sensitive area of the retina and is responsible for its nourishment.

Magnetic resonance imaging (MRI): A noninvasive diagnostic technique that can provide information on the form and function of internal tissue and organs of the body.

Malaise: A generalized feeling of discomfort.

Malignancy: A *neoplasm* or tumor replicating out of control and invading tissue and causing damage to that tissue.

Mast cell: A granulocyte found in tissue. The contents of the mast cells, along with those of basophils, are responsible for the symptoms of allergy.

Melanoma: A cancer made up of pigmented skin cells.

Memory cell: A T cell that has been exposed to a specific antigen and is able thereafter to proliferate upon repeated exposure to the same antigen.

Meningitis: Inflammation of one (or more than one) of the three membranes (meninges) covering the brain and spinal cord (an *OI*). It may be caused by bacterial or viral infections.

Meningoencephalitis: Inflammation of the brain and spinal cord and their membranes.

Metabolite: Any substance produced by the metabolism or by a metabolic process.

Metastasis: Secondary spread of cancerous tissue to a location distant from the initial cancer; spread is generally through the bloodstream.

Microbe: A minute living organism; microbes include bacteria, protozoa, and fungi.

Milligram (mg): A unit of weight measurement; 1000 ml equal 1 gram (g).

Mitogen: A natural substance that induces the division of cells and can induce cancer-like effects.

Molecule: The smallest amount of a specific chemical that can exist alone.

Monoclonal antibody: An antibody produced by a single cell or its identical progeny, specific to a given antigen. Monoclonal antibodies are useful as tools for identifying specific protein molecules.

Monocyte: A large white blood cell that acts as a scavenger, capable of destroying invading bacteria or other foreign material. It is a precursor to the *macrophage*.

Mucocutaneous: Concerning or pertaining to *mucous membranes* and the skin.

Mucosal tissue: The tissue that lines the moist cavities of the body that open to the body surface, in particular the mouth, vagina, and rectum.

Mucous membrane: A moist layer of tissue that lines body cavities or passages that have an opening to the external world, e.g., the lining of the mouth, nostrils, vagina, or anus.

Natural killer cell (NK cell): A large, granular lymphocyte that attacks and destroys tumor cells and infected body cells. The cells are known as "natural" killers because they attack without first having to recognize specific antigens.

Necrolysis: Separation or scaling off of tissue due to necrosis (localized tissue death).

Neoplasm: An abnormal and uncontrolled growth of tissue; a tumor.

Neuralgia: A sharp, shooting pain along a nerve pathway.

Neuron: A nerve cell. Viewed microscopically, a neuron is seen to be composed of three parts: *dendrites* with receptor sites that receive information from other cells, a *cell body* that integrates the information from all the receptor sites, and an *axon* that travels sometimes many feet and from which a neurotransmitter is released to pass on information. Sometimes axons and cell bodies can have receptor sites as well.

Neuropathy: Any abnormal, degenerative, or inflammatory state of the peripheral nervous system.

Neutrophil [polymorphonuclear neutrophil (PMN)]: A white blood cell that plays a central role in defense of a host against infection. Neutrophils engulf and kill foreign microorganisms. They are the immune system's primary defense against bacterial infections. The normal range of neutrophils is from 3000 to 7000/ mm^3.

Night sweat: Extreme sweating that happens during sleep. Night sweats are considered a symptom of HIV only when the body is drenched. Slight sweating is not a symptom.

NSAID: Abbreviation for *nonsteroidal anti-inflammatory drug*.

Ocular: Relating to the eye.

Off label: Describes prescription of a drug for conditions other than those intended. Medicaid and Medicare usually will not pay for drugs prescribed "off label."

OI: Abbreviation for *opportunistic infection*.

Oncology: The study of cancer or tumors.

Ophthalmologist: A physician who specializes in treating diseases and refractive errors of the eye.

Opportunistic infection (OI, O/I): An infection that is caused by an agent that is frequently present in our bodies or environment but that causes disease only when there is an alteration from normal, healthy conditions, such as when the immune system becomes depressed.

Optic nerve: The nerve at the back of each eye that carries visual impulses from the retina to the brain.

Oral (p.o.): Taken by mouth as a pill or liquid.

Orphan drug: A drug indicated for rare diseases.

Otitis media: Inflammation of the middle ear.

Pancreas: An organ with a duct into the small intestine, just past the stomach, that secretes proteins ("digestive enzymes") into the intestine to help digest food; also secretes insulin.

Pancreatic: Related to the pancreas.

Pancytopenia: Deficiency of all cellular elements of the blood.

Pandemic: Referring to an epidemic disease of widespread prevalence.

Papilledema: Swelling of the optic nerve caused by increased pressure within the brain; usually presents a minor, transient visual loss.

Paresthesia: A sensation of prickling, tingling, or creeping of the skin that has no objective cause.

Parvovirus: A small virus that is present in about 50% of the population and causes bone marrow failure in immunodeficient people. It may cause aplastic anemia in people with AIDS.

Pathogen: Any disease-producing microorganism or material.

PCP: Abbreviation for *Pneumocystis carinii pneumonia*.

Pelvic inflammatory disease (PID): A condition affecting women that is caused by the spread of infection from the vagina to the pelvic cavity. Most often applies to gonorrhea infections.

Phagocytosis: The process of ingestion and destruction of a virus or other foreign matter by phagocytes (monocytes/macrophages).

Phlebotomy: An incision into a vein for the purpose of drawing blood.

Placebo: An inactive substance against which investigational treatments are compared for efficacy. In placebo-controlled drug studies, a placebo is given to one group of patients, while the drug being tested is given to another group. The results obtained in the two groups are then compared.

Plasma: A fluid in which blood cells and nutritive substances are circulated in the body. It also serves to remove waste products of metabolism from organs and to facilitate chemical communication between different portions of the body.

Plasma cell: A large antibody-producing cell that develops from a *B cell*.

Platelet: A disk-shaped element of the blood, smaller than a red or white blood cell. Platelets are critical for blood clotting and sealing off wounds.

Platelet count: The number of platelets in blood. The normal count is 200,000–300,000 platelets/mm^3.

Pneumocystis carinii pneumonia (PCP or interstitial plasma cell pneumonia): A lung infection seen in immunosuppressed people. Once thought to be caused by a protozoan, it now appears to be fungal in origin.

Prophylactic: A drug that helps to prevent a disease before it occurs.

Prophylaxis: A treatment intended to preserve health and prevent the spread of disease (e.g., aerosolized pentamidine has shown effectiveness as a prophylaxis against *PCP*).

Protein: An organic compound made up of amino acids. Proteins are one of the major constituents of plant and animal cells.

PWA: Abbreviation for *person* (or *people*) *with AIDS*.

Quinolone antibiotic: One of a class of synthetic, broad-spectrum antibacterial agents that includes ciprofloxacin and sparfloxacin.

Radiation therapy: A treatment for malignant disease using radiation.

Recombinant: Produced by genetic engineering.

Reiter's syndrome: An autoimmune disease that sometimes appears in young men with AIDS.

Remission: The lessening of the severity or duration of outbreaks, or the abatement of symptoms altogether over a period of time.

Renal: Pertaining to the kidneys.

Resistance: The ability of an organism to overcome the inhibiting effects of a drug. The organism is said to be "resistant" to that drug.

Retina: The innermost covering of the eyeball, on which the image is formed.

Retinal disease: Any disease of the retina, the innermost layer of the eyeball.

Retinitis: Inflammation of the retina, linked in AIDS to *CMV* infection. Untreated, it can lead to blindness.

Retinopathy: Any noninflammatory disease of the retina.

Retrovir: See *Zidovudine (AZT)*.

Retrovirus: A class of viruses that copy genetic material using RNA as a template for making DNA. (HIV is a retrovirus.)

Reverse transcriptase: A retroviral enzyme that is capable of copying RNA into DNA, an essential step in the life cycle of HIV.

Rheumatoid arthritis: A chronic systemic disease primarily of the joints with inflammation, atrophy, deformity, and immobilization (an *OI*). The cause is unknown, but autoimmune mechanisms and viral infection are suspected. It is included here as an immune system disease.

Ribonucleic acid (RNA): A complex nucleic acid responsible for the transmission of genetic information in retroviruses. In cells, RNA transfers the genetic information contained in DNA to proteins.

Safer sex: A system of classifying specific sexual activities according to their risk of transmitting HIV; safer sex guidelines are used by people to avoid high-risk behavior without having to give up sexual activity. Those acts that are defined as "safe" involve no exchange of body fluids.

Salivary gland: One of the tissue structures in the mouth and gastrointestinal tract that produce proteins ("digestive enzymes") that help to digest food.

Salmonella: A genus of bacteria that causes gastroenteritis in humans (an *OI*).

Sarcoma: A malignant tumor of the skin and soft tissue.

Sclera: The white portion of the eyeball.

Scleroderma: An autoimmune illness with hardening and shrinking of the connective tissues of parts of the body, including the skin, heart, esophagus, kidneys, and lungs (an opportunistic infection). Pigmented patches of skin may occur. It is an immune system disease.

Seroconversion: Change in a person's antibody status from negative to positive.

Seropositive: Having manufactured antibodies against the HIV infection.

Shigellosis: The disease produced by infection with *Shigella*. The digestive disturbances caused by *Shigella* can range from mild diarrhea to severe or even fatal dysentery.

Shingles: See *herpes zoster*.

Spleen: A lymphoid organ in the abdominal cavity that is an important center for immune system activities.

STD: Abbreviation for *sexually transmitted disease*.

Stem cell: The type of cell from which all blood cells derive. Bone marrow is rich in stem cells.

Steroid: Any of numerous compounds that include sterol-like substances, certain hormones, D vitamins, and some carcinogenic substances. Steroids are often used to reduce inflammation in the body.

Streptococcus: A genus of cocci (bacteria) that causes infections in the throat, respiratory system, and skin. Improperly treated, the infection can lead to disease in the heart, joints, and kidneys.

Subcutaneous: Beneath or introduced beneath the skin (e.g., subcutaneous injections).

Suppressor T cell (T8, CD8): One of a subset of *T cells* that halt antibody production and other immune responses.

Symptom: Any perceptible, subjective change in the body or its functions that indicates disease or phases of disease, as reported by the patient.

Syncytium: A dysfunctional multicellular clump formed by fusion.

Syndrome: A group of symptoms and diseases that together are characteristic of a specific condition.

Syphilis: A venereal disease caused by the spirochete *Treponema pallidum*. Some scientific and popular theoreticians believe that AIDS is caused by either the treponema associated with syphilis or a related treponema. Syphilis is an infectious, chronic, sexually transmitted disease caused by a bacterium and characterized by lesions that may involve any organ or tissue. It usually exhibits skin manifestations, relapses are frequent, and it may exist without symptoms for years.

T cell (T lymphocyte): A thymus-derived white blood cell that participates in a variety of cell-mediated immune reactions. Three fundamentally different types of T cells are recognized: *T helper*, *T killer*, and *T suppressor*; each of these types in turn has many subdivisions.

T helper cell: One of a subset of T cells that carry the T4 marker and are essential for turning on antibody production, activating cytotoxic T cells, and initiating other immune responses.

Thrush: A *candida* infection of the mouth or throat characterized by the formation of white patches and ulceration of the affected tissues, usually forming a white curdlike deposit on the tongue, cheeks, and palate that may cause severe discomfort. It is caused by infection with *Candida albicans*, and the condition is known technically as *candidiasis*.

Tissue: A group of cells that act together for a specific purpose.

Titer or titre: A laboratory measurement of the amount (or concentration) of a given component in a solution.

T killer cell: A type of white blood cell that kills foreign organisms after being activated by the *T helper cells*.

Toxicity: The extent, quality, or degree of being poisonous or harmful to the body.

T suppressor cell: A type of white blood cell that helps regulate the body's response to an infection.

Tuberculosis (TB): An infection caused by *Mycobacterium tuberculosis*. Treatment consists of the administration of a combination of bacterial drugs, usually for at least nine months. Immunization with BCG (bacillus calmette-Guérin) gives some protection in susceptible people; however, it renders the person permanently positive to tuberculin tests in the future. TB among *PWAs* is not uncommon.

Uric acid: A product of protein digestion that is eliminated from the body in urine.

Vaccine: A substance that contains antigenic components from an infectious organism. By stimulating an immune response (but not disease), it protects against subsequent infection by that organism.

Vaginal candidiasis: Infection in the vagina with *Candida albicans*, the fungus that causes *thrush*. Presents with pain, itching, redness, and white patches in the vaginal wall. Much more common and more difficult to treat in women with HIV infection; felt by some physicians to represent an opportunistic infection when it develops in women with HIV infection.

Vascular: Pertaining to blood vessels.

Viral culture: A laboratory method for growing viruses.

Virology: The study of viruses and viral disease.

Virus: The smallest known infectious organism. Viruses are a group of infectious agents characterized by their inability to reproduce outside of a living cell. A virus may subvert the host cell's normal functions, causing the cell to behave in a manner determined by the virus. Viruses are unable to live or multiply outside of a host cell, since most do not possess the means to synthesize protein.

Visceral: Pertaining to the major internal organs.

Wasting syndrome: A condition characterized by involuntary weight loss of more than 10% of *baseline* body weight plus either chronic diarrhea or chronic weakness and fever for more than 30 days, when these conditions cannot be explained by any illness other than HIV infection.

Western blot: A test for the presence of specific antibodies, more accurate than the *ELISA* test.

White blood cell: Any of many types of cells that protect the body against foreign substances such as disease-producing microorganisms. They are part of the immune system.

Zidovudine (ZUD): An *antiviral* drug; the first drug developed for use against HIV infection and AIDS. Formerly known as AZT.

Zovirax: See *acyclovir (ACV)*.

Appendix

A

Phone Resources

Alabama	1-800-228-0469	Montana	1-800-233-6668
Alaska	1-800-478-2437	Nebraska	1-800-782-2437
Arizona	1-602-420-9396	Nevada	1-800-842-2437
Arkansas	1-800-448-8305	New Hampshire	1-800-872-8909
California	1-800-367-2437	New Jersey	1-800-624-2377
New Mexico	1-800-545-2437	Colorado	1-800-252-2437
New York	1-800-541-2437	Connecticut	1-800-342-AIDS
North Carolina	1-800-342-AIDS	Delaware	1-800-422-0429
North Dakota	1-800-472-2180	District of Columbia	1-202-332-2437
Ohio	1-800-332-2437	Florida	1-800-352-2437
Oklahoma	1-800-535-2437	Georgia	1-800-551-2728
Oregon	1-800-777-2437	Hawaii	1-800-922-1313
Pennsylvania	1-800-662-6080	Idaho	1-208-345-2277
Puerto Rico	1-800-765-1010	Illinois	1-800-243-2437
Rhode Island	1-800-726-3010	Indiana	1-800-848-2437
South Carolina	1-800-322-2437	Iowa	1-800-445-2437
South Dakota	1-800-592-1861	Kansas	1-800-232-0040
Kentucky	1-800-654-2437	Texas	1-800-299-2437
Louisiana	1-800-922-4379	Utah	1-800-366-2437
Maine	1-800-851-2437	Vermont	1-800-882-2437
Maryland	1-800-638-6252	Virginia	1-800-533-4138
Massachusetts	1-800-235-2331	Virgin Islands	1-809-773-2437
Michigan	1-800-872-2437	Washington	1-800-272-2437
Minnesota	1-800-248-2437	West Virginia	1-800-642-8244
Mississippi	1-800-537-0851	Wisconsin	1-800-334-2437
Missouri	1-800-533-2437	Wyoming	1-800-327-3577

Appendix

B

Publications

AIDS Treatment News
John S. James
PO Box 411256
San Francisco, CA 94141

$100/year or $60/6 months; write for sliding scale. Covers current drug trials, interviews, very active.

Body Positive
51-B Philbeach Gardens
London SW5 9EB, U.K.

Inquire for subscription. Part of its appeal is that it carries news that is not necessarily available in United States publications. Monthly.

Body Positive
2095 Broadway
Suite 306
New York, NY 10023

According to an item in "Positively Aware," this is a "monthly newsletter for HIV-positive people, available in Spanish on a limited basis. Voluntary contributions accepted." Is obviously not the same as the British "Body Positive."

Bulletin of Experimental Treatments for AIDS
San Francisco AIDS Foundation
BETA Subscription Department
PO Box 426182
San Francisco, CA 94142

$45 or ability to pay for PWAs, $90 for organizations, free for San Francisco residents.

Critical Path AIDS Project
% Kiyoshi Kuromiya
2062 Lombard Street
Philadelphia, PA 19146

Free to PWAs, $50 to others. Along with specific medical news, social concerns are addressed; some excerpts of interest from other publications. Monthly.

I Heard It Through the Grapevine
% APLA
6721 Romaine Street
Los Angeles, CA 90038

Ability to pay. Published by Stephen Korsia, an "experimental treatment specialist," on a variable schedule.

Medic Alert
% NAPWA
1413 K Street N.W.
Washington, DC 20005

Free. Combines conventional treatment news and some very solid general articles with other, rather speculative items. Has bad-mouthed the *New England Journal of Medicine* in a "news item." Cosponsored by T2 Medical, Inc.

Notes from the Underground
PWA Health Group of NYC Buyers' Club
150 West 26th Street
Suite 201
New York, NY 10001

$75 to institutions, $35 to others, sliding scale for PWAs. As you'd expect, focus here is on alternative therapies and one step further into "underground" treatments. Published bimonthly.

PI Perspective
% Project rm
1965 Market Street
Suite 220
San Francisco, CA 94103

Sliding scale, inquire. Some content of social import along with highly comprehensive articles about (mostly) alternative therapies. Very energetic. Twice yearly; "briefing papers" available at various other times.

Positively Aware
Test Positively Aware Network, Inc.
1340 West Irving Park
Box 259
Chicago, IL 60613

Although one source is advising people that this is a community-oriented monthly, the issues we've seen are universal in relevance and, as of our June, 1992 file issue, it's a quarterly. Thematic, often characterized as "bright and basic" for the newly diagnosed person with HIV. Write or call (312) 472-6397 to subscribe.

The Positive Woman
P.O. Box 34372
Washington, DC 20043

$75 or sliding scale for PWAs. Presents a mix of conventional and other therapy information, plus reader input, social issues, etc., from a woman's perspective and for an audience that's mostly female. Published at 2-month intervals.

Step Perspective
Seattle Treatment Education Project
127 Broadway East
Suite 200
Seattle, WA 98102

Ability to pay. A mixture of conventional and alternative treatment news, plus general articles for PWA audience. Has earned some good reviews. Three times per year.

Treatment and Data Digest
% ACT UP/New York
135 West 29th Street
New York, NY 10001

$40. Political/activism items accompanied by clinical trials and other medical developments. Said to be one of the most aggressive in obtaining "fast-breaking" developments. One hopes that this arm of ACT UP is in a more stable condition than others seem to be. Twice monthly.

Treatment Issues
% Gay Men's Health Crisis/Medical Information
129 West 20th Street
2nd Floor
New York, NY 10011

$30 for individuals, $50 for organizations, PWAs write and make offer. A good general publication including medical trial news, other advances, and educational features. Issued 10 times/year.

World
% Rebecca Denison
PO Box 11535
Oakland, CA 94611

Sliding scale, inquire. Written for the female audience, covers therapies and research, also addresses political and social issues. Monthly.

References

Chapter 1

Batt, M., 1994. Update on mycobacterial issues for the acquired immune deficiency syndrome era. *Journal of Nursing* 17(4):217–219.

Benedict, S., 1994. Fungal infections associated with malignancies, treatments, and AIDS. *Cancer Nurse* 17(5):411–417.

Bosch, O. et al., 1994. Endoscopic appearance of a duodenal infection by *Mycobacterium avium-intracellulare* in AIDS. *Endoscopy* 26(5):506.

Caiaffa, W. et al., 1994. Drug smoking, Pneumocystis carinii pneumonia, and immunosuppression increase risk of bacterial pneumonia in human immunodeficiency virus–seropositive injection drug users. *American Journal of Respiratory Critical Care Medicine* 150(6 Pt. 1):1493–1498.

Dowler, J. G. et al., 1995. Retinal detachment and herpes virus retinitis in patients with AIDS. *British Journal of Ophthalmology* 79(6):575–580.

Drobniewski, F. A. et al., 1995. Tuberculosis and AIDS. *Journal of Medical Microbiology* 43(2):85–91.

Fong, I. W. et al., 1995. The natural history of progressive multifocal leukoencephalopathy in patients with AIDS. *Clinical Infectious Disease* 20(5):1305–1310.

Fujii, K. et al., 1994. Adrenal insufficiency in a patient with acquired immunodeficiency syndrome. *Endocrinology Journal* 41(1):13–18.

Hanau, L. et al., 1994. *Mycobacterium marinum* infection in a patient with the acquired immunodeficiency syndrome. *New England Journal of Medicine* 54(2):103–105.

Hedges, 1994. Ophthalmoplegia associated with AIDS. *Transactions of the Third Survey of Ophthalmology* 39(1):43–51.

Huebner, R. et al., 1994. Delayed-type hypersensitivity anergy in human immunodeficiency virus–infected persons screened for infection with *Mycobacterium tuberculosis*. *Clinical Infectious Diseases* 19(1): 26–32.

Isaacs, S. et al., 1994. Fulminant reexpansion pulmonary edema in a patient with AIDS. *Annals of Emergency Medicine* 24(5):975–977.

Jones, B. et al., 1994. A prospective of antituberculosis therapy in patients with human immunodeficiency virus infection. *American Journal of Respiratory Critical Care Medicine* Dec:150.

Kimura, S. et al., 1994. Symmetrical external capsule lesions in a patient with herpes simplex encephalitis. *Neuropediatrics* 25(3):162–164.

Khoo, S. et al., 1994. Invasive aspergillosis in patients with AIDS. *Clinical Infectious Diseases* 19(Suppl 1):S41–S48.

Miralles, E. et al., 1994. Mucocutaneous leishmaniasis and HIV. *Dermatology* 189(3):275–277.

Miralles, G., 1994. Disseminated *Nocardia farcinica* infection in an AIDS patient. *European Journal of Clinical Microbiology and Infectious Disease* 13(6):497–500.

Mitchell, S. et al., 1994. Vitreous fluid sampling and viral genome detection for the diagnosis of viral retinitis in patients with AIDS. *Journal of Medical Virology* 43(4):336–340.

Musiani, M. et al., 1994. Rapid diagnosis of cytomegalovirus encephalitis in patients with AIDS using in situ hybridisation. *Journal of Clinical Pathology* 47(10):886–891.

Peavy, G. et al., 1994. Verbal memory performance of patients with human immunodeficiency virus infection: Evidence of subcortical dysfunction. *Clinical Neuropsychology* 16(4):508–523.

Perazella, M. et al., 1994. Acute nonspecific illness in an AIDS patient with dysphagia. *Hospital Practice* 29(11):39, 43, 47.

Portegies, P., 1994. AIDS dementia complex: A review. *Acquired Immune Deficiency Syndrome* 7(Suppl. 2):S38–S48.

Revello, M. et al., 1994. Diagnosis of human cytomegalovirus infection of the nervous system by pp65 detection in polymorphonuclear leukocytes of cerebrospinal fluid from AIDS patients. *Journal of Infectious Diseases* 170(5):1275–1279.

Richter, C. et al., 1994. Clinical features of HIV-seropositive and HIV-seronegative patients with tuberculous pleural effusion in Dar es Salaam, Tanzania. *Chest* 106(5):1471–1475.

Vaughan Jones, S., 1994. Chronic verrucous varicella-zoster infection in a patient with AIDS. *Clinical Dermatology* 19(4):327–329.

Wang, C. Y. et al., 1995. Skin cancers associated with acquired immunodeficiency syndrome. *Mayo Clinic* 70(8):766–772.

Yee, J. et al., 1995. Gastrointestinal manifestations of AIDS. *Gastroenterology Clinics of North America* 24(2):413–434 (45 references).

Chapter 2

Rey, D. et al., 1995. Differences in HIV testing, knowledge and attitudes in pregnant women who deliver and those who terminate. *AIDS Care* 7(Suppl. 1):S39–46.

Yasuda, S. et al., 1994. Studies on the HIV-specific IgA antibodies in sera and saliva. *International Conference on AIDS* 10(1):228.

Chapter 3

Chapman, K. et al., 1995. Testing patients for HIV before surgery: The views of doctors performing surgery. *AIDS Care* 7(2):125–128.

Levine, C., 1995. Orphans of the HIV epidemic: Unmet needs in six US cities. *AIDS Care* 7(Suppl. 1):S57–S62.

Phillips, K. A. et al., 1995. HIV counseling and testing: Research and policy issues. *AIDS Care* 7(2):115–124.

World Health Organization global AIDS statistics, 1995. *AIDS Care* 7(2): 244–248.

Wortley, P. M. et al., 1995. HIV testing patterns: Where, why, and when were persons with AIDS tested for HIV? *AIDS* 9(5):487–492.

Chapter 4

Hu, D. J. et al., 1995. Characteristics of persons with late AIDS diagnosis in the United States. *American Journal of Preventive Medicine* 11(2):114–119.

Levy, L. A., 1995. History and epidemiology of acquired immune deficiency syndrome. *Journal of the American Podiatric Medical Association* 85(7):346–351.

News update on AIDS in men who have sex with men, 1995. *American Family Physician* 52(2):667.

Sultan, J. et al., 1994. Human immunodeficiency virus infection presenting as pancytopenia in an infant. *American Journal of Pediatric Hematology and Oncology* 16(4):334–337.

Weinstock, H. S. et al., 1995. Trends in HIV seroprevalence among persons attending sexually transmitted disease clinics in the United States, 1988–1992. *Journal of Acquired Immune Deficiency Syndrome and Human Retrovirology* 9(5):514–522.

Chapter 5

Arribas, J. R. et al., 1995. Level of cytomegalovirus (CMV) DNA in cerebrospinal fluid of subjects with AIDS and CMV infection of the central nervous system. *Journal of Infectious Diseases* 172(2):527–531.

Bennett, C. et al., 1994. A rapid preadmission method for predicting inpatient course of disease for patients with HIV-related Pneumocystis carinii pneumonia. *American Journal of Respiratory Critical Care Medicine* 150(6 Pt. 1):1503–1507.

Coward, D. D., 1995. The lived experience of self-transcendence in women with AIDS. *Journal of Obstetrics and Gynecological Neonatal Nursing* 24(4):314–318.

Galli, L. et al., 1995. Onset of clinical signs in children with HIV-1 perinatal infection. *AIDS* 9(5):455–461.

Schmidt, J., 1995. Crossing the black ocean: For many AIDS patients, the journey toward death is too long. *American Journal of Nursing* 95(8):72.

Tsukada, S. et al., 1994. Role of Brutan's tyrosine kinase in immunodeficiency. *Current Opinion in Immunology* 6(4):623–630.

Whitson, B. et al., 1994. Fatal mycobacterial infection in a 32-year-old man with AIDS. *New England Journal of Medicine* 106(5):1577–1579.

Chapter 6

James, J. S., 1995. Protease inhibitors: Merck plans larger trials, expanded access. *AIDS Treatment News.* Mar 24, No. 219:6.

James, J. S., 1995. FDA reform in Congress: AIDS community absent. Food and Drug Administration. *AIDS Treatment News.* Apr. 7, No. 220:4–5.

Lewis, D. et al., 1994. AIDS immune response following oral administration of cholera toxin B subunit to HIV-1-infected UK and Kenyan subjects. *New England Journal of Medicine* 8(6):779–785.

Merck protease inhibitor MK-639—trial cities announced, 1995. *AIDS Treatment News.* Apr. 7, No. 220:1–2.

Nageswaran, A. et al., 1994. Bilateral spontaneous pneumothorax in AIDS—successful treatment with talc pleurodesis following failure with tetracycline sclerotherapy. *International Journal of STD and AIDS* 5(4):296–298.

O'Brien, R., 1994. Drug-resistant tuberculosis: Etiology, management and prevention. *Respiratory Infection* 9(2):104–112.

Okwera, A. et al., 1994. Randomised trial of thiacetazone and rifampicin-containing regimens for pulmonary tuberculosis in HIV-infected Ugandans. *Makerere University–Case Western University Research* 344(8933):1323.

Patel, A. et al., 1994. Disseminated cutaneous nocardiosis as a presenting illness of HIV infection. *New England Journal of Medicine* 161(10): 609–611.

Scaglia, M. et al., 1994. Effectiveness of aminosidine (Paromomycin) sulfate in chronic cryptosporidium diarrhea in AIDS patients: An open, uncontrolled, prospective clinical trial. *Journal of Infectious Diseases* 170(5):1349–1350.

Sewell, D. et al., 1994. Neuroleptic treatment of HIV-associated psychosis. *Neuropsychopharmacology* 10(4):223–229.

Viswanathan, R. et al., 1994. Stereotoxic brain biopsy in AIDS patients: Does it contribute to patient management? *British Journal of Neurosurgery* 8(3):307–311.

Wallace, M. et al., 1994. Invasive aspergillosis in patients with AIDS. *Clinical Infectious Diseases* 19(1):222.

Chapter 7

Baker, J., 1989. A racist ambush in NY. *Newsweek*, September 4.

Baker, J., 1991. Battling the bias. *Newsweek*, November 29.

Block, A. 1991. Sexual amnesty. *Mother Jones*, July/August.

Bloom, J. (Ed.), 1987. *The Bible*, Chelsea House: New York.

Boast, N. et al., 1994. Homosexual erotomania and HIV infection. *British Journal of Psychiatry* 164(6):842–846.

Clift, E., 1992. The right wing's cultural warriors. *Newsweek*, July 17.

Clift, E., 1992. How the candidates play to the gays. *Newsweek*, September 14.

Cohen, J. 1995. Women: Absent term in the AIDS research education. *Science* 269(5225):777–780.

Dahir, M., 1992. Coming out of the barrel. *The Progressive*, June.

Ehrenreich, B., 1992. Making sense of la difference. *Time*, January 20.

Frenkel, L. M. et al., 1995. Effects of zidovudine use during pregnancy on resistance and vertical transmission of human immunodeficiency virus type I. *Clinical Infectious Diseases* 20(5):1321–1326.

Kail, B. L. et al., 1995. Needle-using practices within the sex industry. *American Journal of Drug and Alcohol Abuse* 21(2):241–255.

Kalichman, S. C. et al., 1995. Context framing to enhance HIV-antibody-testing messages targeted to African American women. *Health Psychology* 14(3):247–254.

Kalichman, S. and Henderson, M., 1991. MMPI profile subtypes of non-incarcerated child molesters: A cross validation study. *Criminal Justice and Behavior*, December.

Kinsey, A., 1948. *Sexual Behavior in the Human Male*. W. B. Saunders: Philadelphia.

Lautmann, R., 1990. Categorization in concentration camps as a collective fate: A comparison of homosexuals, Jehovah's Witnesses and political prisoners. *Journal of Homosexuality*, January.

Leonard, A., 1990. Report from the legal front. *The Nation*, July 2.

Minkowitz, D., 1992. It's still open season on gays. *The Nation*, March 23.

Mohr, J., 1992. *Gays/Justice: A Study of Ethics, Society and Law*. Columbia University Press: New York.

Noll, M., 1992. Theology, science, politics: What Darwin meant. *Christian Century*, August 26.

Nyamathi, A. et al., 1995. Psychosocial predictors of AIDS risk behavior and drug use behavior in homeless and drug addicted women of color. *Health Psychology* 14(3):265–273.

Rist, D., 1990. Global gay bashing. *Utne Reader*, November/December.

Ryan, L. 1995. "Going public" and "watching sick people"—the clinic setting as a factor in the experiences of gay men participating in AIDS clinical trials. *AIDS Care* 7(2):147–158.

Spinillo, A. et al., 1994. Clinical and microbiological characteristics of symptomatic vulvovaginal candidiasis in HIV-seropositive women. *New England Journal of Medicine* 70(4):268–272.

United Nations Chronicle, 1990. The 44th General Assembly: A turning point in UN history, March.

Van de Perre, P., 1995. Postnatal transmission of human immunodeficiency virus Type 1: The breast-feeding dilemma. *American Journal of Obstetrics and Gynecology* 173(2):483–487.

Walter, E. B. et al., 1995. Maternal acceptance of voluntary human immunodeficiency virus antibody testing during the newborn period with the Guthrie Card. *Pediatric Infectious Disease Journal* 14(5):376–381.

Zeman, N., 1992. No special rights for gays: Colorado voters pass anti-gay amendment. *Newsweek*, November 23.

Chapter 8

Bletzer, K. V., 1995. Use of ethnography in the evaluation and targeting of HIV/AIDS education. *AIDS Education and Prevention* 7(2):178–191.

Fanburg, J. T. et al., 1995. Student opinions of condom distribution at a Denver, Colorado, high school. *Journal of School Health* 65(5):181–185.

Fisher, W. A. et al., 1994. Understanding and promoting AIDS-preventive behavior: Insights from the theory of reasoned action. *Health Psychology* 14(3):255–264.

Gold, R., 1995. Why we need to rethink AIDS education for gay men. *AIDS Care* 7(Suppl. 1):S11–S19.

Kann, L. et al., 1995. Youth risk behavior surveillance—United States, 1993. *Journal of School Health* 65(5):163–171.

Latman, N. S. et al., 1994. Behavioral risk of human immunodeficiency virus/acquired immunodeficiency syndrome in the university student community. *Sexually Transmitted Diseases* 22(2):104–109.

Lifson, A. R., 1995. Preventing AIDS: Have we lost our way? *Lancet* 346(8970):262–263.

Oakley, A. et al., 1995. Behavioural interventions for HIV/AIDS prevention. *AIDS* 9(5):479–486.

Ogden, J. et al., 1993. Beliefs about condoms in 12/13 and 16/17 year olds. *AIDS Care* 7(2):205–210.

Stevenson, H. C. et al., 1995. Culturally sensitive AIDS education and perceived AIDS risk knowledge: Reaching the "know-it-all" teenager. *AIDS Education and Prevention* 7(2):134–144.

Index